Mommy Fabulous

Complete Pregnancy Fitness and Nutrition Guide

Designed to Deliver
a Fabulous Postpartum Figure

DANIELLE FEDERICO, M.P.H.

The information in this book should not be used instead of medical advice. You should speak to your doctor about your health, especially about things that may need diagnosis or medical attention. Women should seek prenatal care as soon as they know they are pregnant and continue until the baby is born.

For inquiries please go to
www.dani-fabulous.com

ISBN-10: 1466427892
ISBN-13: 978-1466427891

Cover photographed by Brodie Jayne
Interior fitness photography by Devin Giannoni

Dedication

To my friend and maternity workout partner Jayme who encouraged me to write a book on my maternity workout program

and to

my daughter Talia who has changed my life in immeasurable ways

CONTENTS

I'm Pregnant!

I had started feeling unusually tired by late afternoon. After two weeks of fatigue, I made an appointment with my doctor to see if I had Mono or some nasty bug that was draining my energy. I knew the doctor would first ask if I was pregnant because they ask that every time you go to the doctor…even if you are there because you have a splinter stuck in your hand. I knew I wasn't, but I was not going to pay the expense of a lab test when at-home tests are so much cheaper. It was eight pm when I got back from the gym and decided to take a pregnancy test just so I could tell the doctor that I knew for sure I wasn't pregnant. I jumped in the shower and did a face mask; it wasn't until I finished brushing my teeth that I remembered to check the test. I was honestly confused when I saw the plus sign because I wasn't pregnant. I even grabbed the box to make sure that a plus sign means positive. (Heck, maybe a plus sign means something else in some foreign country where this test was manufactured.) According to the box, a plus sign universally means positive no matter what country you are in. BUT it also said results need to be read within three minutes and at least ten minutes had passed before I checked it. So I drank a glass of water and took the test again. This time I waited in the bathroom for the three minutes to make sure the testing procedure was accurate; I mean I really didn't want the drama of another false positive. + again! What? I mean…WHAT? My doctor confirmed it the next day. I was pregnant. I was also less than ecstatic.

I was definitely not ready for this. I was very into my career and social life. For vain reasons, I did not want to be pregnant. Having an unexpected child is one thing, I mean, if my husband was pregnant I could deal with the surprise, but I did not want to be the one to carry and deliver this baby. I thought about how a caterpillar forms a cocoon and then emerges as a butterfly. This baby was going to emerge from this pregnancy as a beautiful creature that would learn to soar. But where did that leave me? The old remnants of a used cocoon? Of course some of my fears were purely vain, okay well maybe more like most of them. But my husband was not going to have to sacrifice his youthful figure. He would not be left with the scares of childbearing in the form of a pooch belly or stretch marks. It simply isn't fair that society judges women so harshly about their looks when childbearing ruins them. I was not going to let pregnancy dictate how I looked after delivery. I was going to be the master of my own figure…even if my body was currently being occupied by another person. I too wanted to emerge from this pregnancy as a new born person. So I decided that is what was going to happen. I decided I had to become Mommy Fabulous.

Whether it is socially or culturally just, most women feel a desire to look fit and sexy. I don't know anyone who is striving to look overweight and frumpy. While physical appearance may not be a top concern during pregnancy, it usually is a concern that can lead to self esteem issues after pregnancy. While pregnant, I found few resources that actually help pregnant and postpartum women achieve the physical look they want. Most of the time prenatal programs are geared toward providing some level of activity so that the pregnant woman does not live out her nine months as caged veal. But low intensity, non-specific target activities do not keep a pregnant woman fit or prepare her for childbirth or make postpartum recovery any easier. Successfully recovering from an abdominal trauma like giving birth takes some specific techniques that I feel are widely ignored during pregnancy and then become important postpartum- when you don't know how to do them and don't have time to learn them. Thus I engineered a workout plan that takes into account the abilities and weaknesses of the pregnant body as well as the common discomforts and side effects, pairing them with activities that mitigate these effects and maximize your ability to emerge from pregnancy with a more toned, sculpted body than you went in with. I looked at childbirth as an abdominal trauma injury from a physical rehabilitation standpoint and incorporated exercises into the pregnancy program that will speed up your postpartum recovery time. It worked for me and I have been training pregnant clients ever since, showing them how to become Mommy Fabulous.

That's me on the cover six months after giving birth. I am pretty proud of the picture, but it is important to me that you know I did not look like that before I had Talia. Everyone complains about how pregnancy wrecks your body and all you have to look forward to are sagging breasts and stretch marks. Sadly, it is a reality for many women. Some women tell us how we should embrace our new postpartum, albeit misshapen, figures. I was not about that. Surviving pregnancy became my goal. Pregnancy does not have wreck your body if you don't let it. In fact, you can look better than you did before giving birth. The window of opportunity is small, but it is the chance of a lifetime. By eating well and exercising in a specific way you will be able to make safe fitness gains and set yourself up for a quick recovery. You can safely remodel your figure while you are pregnant and while you recover from your pregnancy, emerging on the scene as Mommy Fabulous like you never thought possible.

Pregnancy is an amazing and exciting, if not a bit scary, journey you are experiencing. It is the perfect time to make lifestyle changes and get control of your fitness. When you are pregnant you have the motivation to make serious changes. To me, that means forming health habits. Exercise offers tons of amazing benefits, with little risk, for pregnant women. Yet, only 16% of pregnant women get enough physical activity to meet guideline suggestions.* (Most non-pregnant people don't get enough physical activity, either.) We mothers-to-be are not necessarily to blame. In this era of health awareness, prevention focused medicine and female empowerment, somehow pregnancy has still become accepted as a nine month excuse for gluttony and laziness. Letting yourself go during pregnancy can end up being a lifetime uphill struggle for you. As a personal trainer and nutritional counselor, many clients come to me saying that ever since they had a baby their stomach has never looked the way they want it to. When asked how long ago they delivered, some say ten years. I don't want you to struggle with your body for a decade. I want every woman to experience the Mommy Fabulous fitness and nutrition program and recover from pregnancy looking great and feeling good. I'll provide the tools, you provide the commitment!

*Petersen, A. *Medicine & Science in Sports & Exercise*, October 2005; vol 37: pp 1748-1753. News release, Saint Louis University.

Chapter 1

Eating Safely

The time to assess your eating habits is now. Prior to becoming pregnant, nutrition may not have been a priority for you, maybe it has been. Do you love cooking or hate it? Does your spouse do all the grocery shopping or do you share the responsibility? No matter how your life has operated with regards to food, you should take this opportunity to make healthy nutritional changes that will benefit you and your family for the rest of your life. I will show you how to do this with the Mommy Fabulous style of eating in the following chapters.

Before I can show you how to eat Mommy Fabulous style, I first need to address the foods that are dangerous for a pregnant woman to consume. While you are pregnant, your immune system is working at less than optimum for a few adaptive reasons. While your immune system is in this depressed state you are more susceptible to getting sick from colds, flu and foodborne infection. Be sure to get a flu shot if you are pregnant during flu season.

Some of the foods you may have enjoyed before pregnancy will now pose a food poisoning risk to you and your baby, for three reasons. First, you may not have become ill in the past when exposed to these risks because your immune system was sufficient to handle the infectious agent. While pregnant however, your immune system is weaker than when you are not. Second, if you get food poisoning while pregnant, you can become more ill than you would have when not pregnant, and this can put your baby at risk. Finally, some foodborne infections can cause direct harm to the baby if you are infected by them.

Danger, Danger!

The following foods should not be consumed while pregnant due to the higher risk of infection that could harm your baby.

Soft Cheeses

Imported soft cheeses may contain bacteria called Listeria. Usually this bacterium is not a major health threat, but Listeria has the ability to cross the placenta. The Listeria bacteria can infect the baby or cause blood poisoning, which can be life-threatening and result in a miscarriage. You should avoid soft cheeses such as: Brie, Camembert, Roquefort, Feta, Gorgonzola and Mexican style cheeses, unless they clearly state that they are made from pasteurized milk. The process of pasteurization kills Listeria. Labels that say *raw*, mean not pasteurized. All soft, non-imported cheeses made with pasteurized milk are safe to eat.

Raw or Undercooked Meat

Raw fish, shell fish, poultry and red meat should not be consumed because of the risk of infection with Salmonella, coliform bacteria or Toxoplasmosis. Cook meat until it is no longer pink in the center and wash hands thoroughly after handling raw meat. Only order meat *well done* during pregnancy. When a person is infected with Toxoplasma, there are often no symptoms. However, the Toxoplasma parasite can cross the placenta and infect the baby. Effects on the baby include: premature birth, fever, jaundice, blindness, mental retardation, abnormal head size, seizures, cerebral palsy and deafness. According to the Organization of Teratology Information Services (OTIS), the baby is at the highest risk for severe problems if the infection occurs between weeks 10 and 24.[1]

Raw Eggs

Raw eggs, or any foods that may contain raw eggs, should be avoided due to the risk of infection with Salmonella bacteria. Only buy pasteurized eggs because pasteurization kills Salmonella. There is still a potential for infection when pasteurized eggs are not cooked. Foods that may contain raw eggs include mayonnaise, homemade ice cream, Caesar dressings and Hollandaise sauces. These items usually do not contain raw egg when purchased at a grocery store. However, some restaurants prepare these items fresh and may use raw egg. It is important when dinning out that you ask the server to ask the chef if raw eggs are used and let them know you are pregnant. Don't be embarrassed about doing this, more people ask than you might think. Or you could simply order something else. Avoiding raw eggs means you shouldn't eat raw cookie dough or batter when you are baking.

Unpasteurized Milk or Juice

Unpasteurized milk and juice may also contain Listeria or Toxoplasma. There has been food poisoning outbreaks associated with smoothies made with unpasteurized juice. If you're making a smoothie at home or ordering one at a restaurant, make sure it is made with pasteurized juice. Fresh-squeezed juice sold at fairs, roadside stands, and farmer's markets or in some restaurants may not be pasteurized. Milk and juices that are pasteurized are safe to drink. Organic milk and juice can still be pasteurized, just check the label. Avoid labels that say *raw*, which means not pasteurized.

Deli Meat

Deli meats can be contaminated with Listeria. Deli meat refers to any packaged or sliced meat. If you enjoy sandwiches, you should eat a grilled chicken breast sandwich or a carver turkey sandwich which will have a piece of chicken or turkey cut from an actual cooked bird, not sliced off a packaged round. If you still don't understand the difference between deli meat and other meat, ask yourself if you see an oven or rotisserie where the meat was cooked or only refrigerators where thin sliced meat is kept. Avoid the later.

Pate

Avoid refrigerated pate or meat spreads as they may contain Listeria bacteria. Canned pate, or shelf-safe meat spreads should be safe to eat.

Smoked Seafood

Refrigerated, smoked seafood can also be contaminated with Listeria. Lox, kippered, nova style, or jerky smoked seafood should be avoided. Canned or shelf-safe smoked seafood can be eaten.

Sprouts

Many outbreaks of food poisoning have been linked to eating raw or lightly cooked sprouts, especially, alfalfa, clover and mung bean sprouts. Bacteria can contaminate sprout seeds. When the sprouts are grown they are contaminated from the inside, so the bacteria can't be washed off.[2] When ordering food at restaurants or delis, make sure to ask for no sprouts and check your food to make sure. Even though I am no longer pregnant, I still avoid sprouts because of contamination issues.

Unwashed Fruit and Vegetables

The Toxoplasma parasite can be found on unwashed fruits and vegetables. Toxoplasma can be on produce whether it is organic or not. Toxoplasma can be found in cat feces, which is often buried in the dirt. If you garden, or grow your own fruit and vegetables, wear gloves to avoid infection. (On a side note, you should not clean your cat's liter box while pregnant.) Make sure you wash your hands, knives and cutting boards so you don't cross contaminate other foods.

How to wash fruit and vegetables[3]

-Thoroughly rinse raw fruits and vegetables, under warm running water before eating or preparing them. Or wash them right when you get home from the market.

-Use a small vegetable brush to remove surface dirt. You can make a little vinegar-water solution or use a produce cleaner, but scrubbing should be enough.

-Don't use soap, detergents, or bleach solutions to wash produce.

-Wash all fruits, including those that require peeling or cutting - like cantaloupe and other melons. Cutting through a rind that has bacteria on it contaminates the inside of the fruit. Peeling a piece of unwashed fruit gets bacteria on your hands and anything you touch.

-Pat fruit and veggies dry with paper towels or a clean towel.

Fish Containing High Mercury Levels

Don't eat Shark, Swordfish, King Mackerel, or Tilefish while pregnant because they contain high levels of mercury.[4] Additionally, fish obtained from local lakes and streams may contain high levels of mercury. These fish include: bluefish, striped bass, salmon, pike, trout, and walleye. These fish are fine from the grocery store because they are monitored. Those caught while on a personal fishing trip may have been exposed to higher mercury levels. Methylmercury fish contamination has been the cause of several epidemics where babies were born with birth defects due to exposure during pregnancy.[4]

Different types of fish accumulate mercury in their bodies to different degrees. Bigger, longer living fish will have higher levels of mercury accumulated in the meat than smaller ones. I am not talking about fish coming from contaminated lakes next to a factory. Fish everywhere are exposed to organic mercury through snow and rain run off which accumulate in streams and the ocean. Mercury is toxic and can not be destroyed by cooking. Methylmercury crosses the placenta and causes many birth defects including blindness, small head size, cerebral palsy, mental retardation, muscle weakness, and seizures.[4]

Here is a list of fish that have the lowest mercury levels compared to other types of fish. If the fish you are considering is not on this list, pass on it while you are pregnant. In fact, mercury contamination of fish is such a serious concern that the Food and Drug Administration (FDA) advises that women who are planning to become pregnant within one year, nursing mothers, and children under the age of six years should also avoid fish that contain high levels of mercury. I don't recommend avoiding fish altogether while pregnant. Fish meat has many benefits including being high in omega-3 fatty acids, vitamins and minerals. The American Heart Association recommends at least two servings of fish per week to help prevent heart disease, lower blood pressure, and reduce the risk of heart attacks and strokes.

Fish Considered Low in Mercury[5]

Enjoy two 6 oz. servings per week

Anchovies	Mackerel (N.Atlantic),Chub (Pacific)
Butterfish	Mullet
Catfish	Oyster
Clam	Perch Ocean
Cod	Salmon
Crab	Sardine
Crawfish	Scallop
Croaker (Atlantic)	Shad American
Flatfish	Shrimp
Haddock (Atlantic)	Squid
Hake	Tilapia
Herring	Trout (Freshwater)
Jacksmelt	Whitefish
Lobster (Spiny)	Whiting

In addition to this list, having a 6 oz. can of chunk, light tuna fish once a month is safe.

Anything That is Not Food

Some pregnant women may crave something that is not food, such as laundry detergent or dirt. This is not your body's way of telling you that you need minerals or that something is wrong with the baby. It is just a weird side effect of pregnancy called pica that some women experience. Talk to your healthcare provider if you crave something that is not food. Do not cave into strange non-food cravings! These items often contain substances that are dangerous to you and your baby.

Caffeine

Most studies, and the American College of Obstetricians and Gynecologists, maintain that consuming 300 mg or less of caffeine a day while pregnant is safe. A 2008 study, however, has found that women who consume 200 mg of caffeine or more per day are twice as likely to have a miscarriage as women who consume no caffeine.[6] Some studies link large caffeine consumption with premature birth, low birth weight, and withdrawal symptoms in infants. Caffeine crosses the placenta and is present in breast milk.[7] The safest thing you can do is avoid caffeine altogether. The next safest thing is to avoid caffeine during the first trimester. Limiting caffeine to 200 mg per day is my most lenient recommendation, but I hope I can convince you to give it up completely.

Caffeine is a stimulant and diuretic. A diuretic causes your body to eliminate water through urination. This is not a good thing, especially while pregnant. During pregnancy it is very easy to become dehydrated and some women have to be hospitalized for dehydration. Diuretics like caffeine can limit your ability to absorb vitamins and minerals from food, or cause vitamin and mineral loss.[8] Caffeine increases stomach acid production which can cause an upset stomach. Now, caffeine may not have that effect on you, but some babies are sensitive to caffeine and become irritable or have difficulty sleeping, even with small amounts of caffeine.[9] Image the effect of caffeine on your unborn baby who can't tell you that you are giving him a stomach ache.

Many people underestimate their caffeine consumption because they only think about how much coffee or soda they drink. More than 200 foods, beverages, and over-the-counter medications contain caffeine! Caffeine is in tea, chocolate, chocolate syrup, chocolate chips, chocolate milk, hot cocoa, energy drinks, herbal products and coffee flavored ice cream, yogurt and candy. A food label that says "decaf" does not mean there is no caffeine. Only "caffeine free" really means there is no caffeine present.

Product	Amount of Caffeine[10]
16 oz. brewed Starbucks coffee	330mg
16 oz. Monster energy drink	160 mg
2 tablets Excedrin extra strength	130 mg
8.3 oz. Red Bull energy drink	80mg
8 oz. Starbucks coffee ice cream	60mg
12 oz. Mountain Dew	55 mg
12 oz. Diet Coke	46mg
8 oz. Green Tea	15-40 mg
1 .55 oz. Hershey chocolate bar	10mg

Herbal Products

Avoid herbal extracts, teas, and pills while pregnant as these products are not regulated by the Food and Drug Administration (FDA). These products are advertised as natural remedies for many medical conditions from common colds to diabetes. Some herbals are even marketed directly for relieving pregnancy symptoms like morning sickness or promoting pregnancy health like "supporting the uterus." The truth is that these promises are made without proper scientific studies to prove the effectiveness of the product or to prove the ingredients are safe for you or your baby. The FDA requires specific scientific studies to establish efficacy and safety of prescription and over-the-counter medications. Additional studies must then be done before a medication can be recommended for use during pregnancy. FDA approved medications must list all ingredients. Herbal products do not undergo any of this scrutiny and the ingredients are not monitored by the FDA. In one bottle you may get very little of the herb and in others too much. Herbal products aren't required to list if they contain caffeine and some have been found to contain contaminants such as lead, prescription drugs, and other substances. If you are buying herbs directly from a natural remedy shop to brew your own tea, you may think they are safer because they are not processed into pill form, but you really have no idea where these herbs have come from, what conditions they have been kept in or what they have been exposed to. Many herbal products stand behind claims that the herb has been used for centuries. This is not proof of effectiveness or safety. I have just given you a list of foods you have eaten your whole life, that now pose risk to your health and your baby's. An herb may help your mood, but it may also cause uterine contractions that can increase your risk of miscarriage or preterm labor. Don't risk it.

Major No - No!

Alcohol

There is no alcohol consumption quantity defined for a pregnant woman. All experts would agree that large amounts of alcohol have been proven to be harmful to a baby, but no actual maximum drink count has been established. My recommendation for a pregnant person is none. Many of us find out we are pregnant a few weeks after conception and find ourselves wracking our brains about how many drinks we may have had in the last week, or whether that party was four weeks ago or six. Don't beat yourself up about this early conception drinking. Now that you know you are pregnant and alcohol is not good for the baby, stop drinking. Drinking alcohol during pregnancy can lead to fetal alcohol syndrome. Babies with fetal alcohol syndrome can have mental retardation, heart defects, and defects of their joints and limbs.

The second reason to cut-out alcohol while pregnant and limit alcohol consumption during the rest of your life is because alcohol slows down your metabolism. That's right. Alcohol is empty calories you are consuming AND it slows down the rate at which you burn calories. A real double whammy! As if that were not enough, alcohol is a diuretic (along with caffeine). Diuretics cause increased urination and therefore water loss. This can result in dehydration. Dehydration is not uncommon during pregnancy. Be sure to drink plenty of water and avoid caffeine and alcohol.

Don't forget to avoid liquor filled chocolates like Amaretto or Grand Marnier or liquor cakes like rum cake. These items will provide only a small exposure to alcohol, but after giving up alcohol, your tolerance will drop off dramatically and even these desserts could leave you feeling sick.

If you are going to a restaurant, hosting a party or want to unwind and enjoy a nice drink, here are a few chic, non-alcoholic options. Mix Pellegrino, Perrier or some other mineral water with lemonade. Float raspberries in it for added sophistication. Put cucumbers, lemon, lime or orange slices in your water. Order a Shirley Temple made with ginger ale; restaurants often substitute cheap, caffeine containing soda instead. Or, order a virgin mixed drink, but beware there is a lot of sugar and calories in a virgin strawberry daiquiri.

Smoking

While technically smoking is not a nutritional issue, cigarettes are put in the mouth so I suppose I should comment. I feel it should be mentioned that smoking is one of the worst decisions you can make with your life and your child's. Women who smoke during pregnancy are more likely to have complications such as vaginal bleeding, miscarriage, stillbirth, and low birthweight babies. Less oxygen and nutrients may reach the fetus which can result in many mental and physical deformities for the child.[11] A 2003 study suggests that babies of mothers who smoke during pregnancy undergo withdrawal-like symptoms after birth similar to those seen in babies of mothers who use some illicit drugs. Babies of smokers appear to be more jittery and difficult to soothe than babies of nonsmokers.[12]

Come on! If you haven't gotten the memo yet, smoking is bad for you. It can cause cancers, lung disease, cardiovascular diseases, osteoporosis, circulatory problems, ulcers, premature aging, low sperm count and impotence. Plus you stink. Even if you don't think you do...you do stink. If you smoke, you have to quit now. Other family members should quit, too. Secondhand smoke is bad for you and the unborn baby. Ask your doctor about where you can find help to quit.

Smoking is a nasty habit that should be avoided throughout a child's life. Chemicals in cigarettes smoked by the mother can be passed to young babies while breastfeeding. Babies who are exposed to secondhand smoke have high rates of lower-respiratory illnesses such as bronchitis, pneumonia and ear infections. Secondhand smoke also increases a child's risk of developing asthma or dying of Sudden Infant Death Syndrome (SIDS).[13] Most smokers say that their parents smoked. Be a role model. Be a parent. Cigarettes aren't food, so they should NOT be in your mouth anyway.

Chapter 2

Vitamins, Supplements and Medication

Prenatal Vitamins

Most physicians and midwives recommend that pregnant women take prenatal vitamins. There are many over-the-counter brands, and some doctors give women prescription prenatal vitamins. How do you decide what to take? First I would like to explain that there is no difference in the quality or safety of vitamins whether they are written and filled by prescription or picked by you and purchased at any pharmacy. Some doctors write prescriptions so you don't have to think about which one to choose. Some insurance companies will pay for prenatal vitamins the way they would pay for blood pressure medication. You should call your own health insurance company and see if prenatal vitamins are covered and ask if they need to be prescribed by a doctor or if you can purchase them and submit the receipt for reimbursement. If your health insurance does not cover prenatal vitamins and your doctor prescribed a certain brand, you should be aware that they may be a lot more expensive because a pharmacy has to fill a prescription. Prescribed prenatal vitamins are no better than the ones sitting on the shelf in front of the pharmacy. You can discuss this with both your doctor and your pharmacist.

Do I really need prenatal vitamins?

I would be irresponsible if I didn't recommend that you take them, but I do want to give you all the facts. According to the American College of Obstetrics and Gynecology, you often can get enough of the nutrients you need if you eat a healthy diet.[14] During pregnancy you need more iron and folic acid to help make extra blood. Please read more about folic acid on page 15. Additional calcium is needed to help build your baby's bones and teeth. You also need extra protein to make blood and build your baby's tissues and muscles. You will not find protein in a vitamin. If cost is an issue, you should check into local organizations that may be able to assist. If you don't look for help, I guarantee it will not find you. You may be able to get by with eating a very healthy diet and using some regular vitamins you already have. Prenatal vitamins do not guarantee a healthy pregnancy and baby. They merely help meet nutritional needs. If you choose not to take prenatal vitamins please follow the nutritional advice in this book carefully.

If you are carrying multiple babies, are underweight, smoke, drink alcohol or lots of caffeine, you should absolutely take prenatal vitamins. Vegetarians and vegans should take prenatal vitamins and may need to take additional iron, vitamin B12, and vitamin D supplements.

My prenatal vitamins make me so nauseous I don't want to take them, do I have to?

Never take your vitamins on an empty stomach which can make you nauseous. Make sure to wash the pills down with a glass of water so they don't stick to your esophagus. If you really can't stand taking them, make sure you are getting enough of the essential nutrients you need while pregnant. The most important additional nutrients you need during pregnancy are:

Nutrient	Prenatal Function	Prenatal Daily Requirement	Sources
Protein	needed for growth of fetal tissue including the brain; needed for growth of breast and uterine tissue; needed to increase maternal blood supply	60-1000 grams	meat, nuts, tofu, beans, seeds
Folic acid	reduces fetal risk of neural tube defects, including spina bifida	600 to 800 micrograms	spinach, peanuts, avocado, orange, kiwi, mango, tomato, melon, oatmeal, beans, lemon, strawberry, grapefruit, cereal
Iron	needed to increase maternal blood volume	27 milligrams	spinach, cereal, oatmeal, meat
Vitamin C	helps with wound healing; tooth and bone development; promotes metabolic processes	85 milligrams	orange, tomato, peppers, kiwi, mango, strawberry, grapefruit, melon, potato
Calcium	helps regulate fluids and helps build fetal bones	1000 milligrams	dairy products, eggs, salmon tofu, almonds

If I take a prenatal vitamin, I don't have to worry about what I eat, right?

Wrong!!!!! One of the most common misconceptions about any type of vitamin is that people think the bottle says it has 100% of the DV (Daily Value) of vitamin A, so they don't think they need any other vitamin A. If this were true, wouldn't we be getting all our nutrients in pill form? Lunch doesn't come in a pill because pill chemistry is not that advanced. Not all pills dissolve completely in the stomach, so not all the vitamins can be absorbed from the pill. Calcium, for example, comes in vitamin pills in the form of calcium carbonate, calcium citrate and tribasic calcium phosphate, among others. The ability of the stomach to absorb each type of calcium is different. You will absorb more calcium from a pill with 100% DV calcium citrate compared to a pill with 100% DV calcium carbonate. But you will definitely NOT get 100% of the daily value from either pill, even if the pills contained 500% of the Daily Value. If you take your multivitamin with a breakfast of sausage, bacon or eggs, the amount of vitamins your body will absorb from the tablet is a lot less than if you took the vitamin with a low fat meal. Vitamins don't provide complex carbohydrates, fiber, water, antioxidants, phytonutrients, protein or fat needed by your body to grow a healthy baby. A prenatal vitamin should be considered as *insurance* for when your best eating efforts aren't good enough. Vitamins are not a substitute for healthy food.

Are prenatal vitamins any different than regular vitamins? Is this just a marketing ploy?

Prenatal vitamins are a little different than regular vitamins. They are usually produced with a vitamin content to meet the daily recommended values for pregnancy. They will have higher levels of iron than regular multivitamins for example. However, marketing does play a role in the price. Just because a vitamin manufacturer has a large add campaign targeted at prenatal health, doesn't mean that the vitamins are any safer or more effective than a cheaper generic brand. Discuss this with your pharmacist.

I keep hearing about Folic Acid, can I only get it from prenatal vitamins?

Folic acid is vitamin B9. Folic acid is probably the most important nutrient you need for pregnancy, and most women do not get enough from their diet. Folic acid reduces the risk of birth defects of the brain and spine. All women of childbearing age should take a 400 microgram vitamin daily. During pregnancy you need 800 milligrams. Folic acid is especially important early in pregnancy. There are many food sources of vitamin B9 including peanuts, spinach, avocados and beans.

Herbal Supplements

Many people opt to take *natural* remedies for aliments as opposed to medication, thinking it is safer. Herbs are drugs just like caffeine, tobacco and medication, even if they are called "natural." After all, medications are discovered and produced based on the medicinal properties of plant extracts or herbs. The reason the list of side effects is so long and scary on medication is because it has been thoroughly studied and legally required. Just because an herb has no label, doesn't mean it has no risks. Herbal extracts, teas and pills are not regulated by the Food and Drug Administration (FDA). For this reason, the label is not legally required to list side effects, or even study whether they exist or not. The FDA requires specific scientific studies to establish efficacy and safety of prescription and over-the-counter medications. Additional studies must then be done before a medication can be recommended for use during pregnancy. These *natural* products can make health claims without proper scientific studies to prove the effectiveness of the product or to prove the ingredients are safe for you or your baby. Many herbal products stand behind claims that the herb has been used for centuries by people in foreign lands. I guarantee that these people have not been taking this herb as a pill for centuries or necessarily while pregnant. Who knows how these people prepared it.

Many people tend to overlook that an herb in a pill, has undergone processing just like medication. The processing that herbs undergo however, is less consistent than medication because herbal manufacturing is not FDA regulated. One bottle may have very little of the herb and in others too much. Herbal products don't have to list if they contain caffeine and some have been found to contain contaminants such as lead, prescription drugs, and other substances.

There have been documented reports of some herbs causing side effects like uterine contractions, which could increase your risk of miscarriage or preterm labor. Some herbs have been removed from the market for causing harm, just like some prescription medications. Even if there are herbs that have been widely used without side effects, most herbal remedies and supplements have not been *proven* to be safe during pregnancy. The American Academy of Pediatrics recommends that pregnant women should limit their consumption of herbal tea. Why risk it? Pregnancy is the time to play it safe when it comes to unstudied, unregulated or experimental supplements or food.

Medication

Medications, both prescription and over-the-counter, cross the placenta and enter the baby's bloodstream. Medication therefore, has the potential to cause birth defects, addiction, or other complications. It is important that you seek medical advice about medications while pregnant. If you go to a physician for a non-pregnancy related matter, and are prescribed medication for any health condition (sinus infection, allergies, plantar wart) be sure to inform the doctor that you are pregnant. Talk to your healthcare provider or pharmacist before taking any over-the-counter medications too.

I am on prescription medication, should I stop taking it now that I am pregnant?

No! Do not stop taking any prescription medication (with the exception of birth control pills) without first talking to your doctor. You should contact your doctor as soon as you realize you are pregnant. Some medicines are safe to take during pregnancy. If you are on a medication that poses a risk, your doctor may be able to recommend switching to a different drug while you are pregnant. In some situations, the risk of not taking a medication may be more harmful to the baby and pregnancy than the potential risk associated with the drug. In these cases, your doctor will weigh the risks of a medication against the effects of not taking them. An example would be chronic hypertension. A woman who has high blood pressure, who becomes pregnant has many treatment options. Her doctor will probably switch her medication to something safer during pregnancy. However, if the woman were to stop taking medication during the pregnancy, her high blood pressure would interfere with the nutritional exchange causing the baby to have low blood pressure. Low blood pressure in the baby can damage the developing kidneys. Another effect of untreated hypertension is a low amount of amniotic fluid. These factors result in what is called intrauterine growth restriction which results in low birth weight babies who have higher risks for various problems.

If I have a prescription to use a drug while pregnant, there is nothing to worry about, right?

Prescription medications labeled "safe for use during pregnancy" can still be harmful if they are abused. Pregnant women who abuse prescription drugs risk overdose and addiction for both themselves and the baby. Prescription medications that are "safe for use during pregnancy" are only safe when used according to the specific dosing directions given by your healthcare provider. And don't mix. If you are on a prescription medication do not take any over-the-counter medications or supplements aside from prenatal vitamins. You don't know what the combined effect will be. Always ask a doctor or pharmacist first.

What can I take while pregnant?

Medicines sold over-the-counter can cause problems during pregnancy. Your pharmacist can give you advice about medicines that are safe for pregnant women. Generally, try not to take any medication unless it is necessary. At the same time, if you have a condition that needs treatment, you don't have to suffer. When taken according to the package directions, the following medications and home remedies have no known harmful effects during pregnancy. This is not a complete list of every safe treatment option, just a list of common and familiar treatments for common conditions. Check with your healthcare provider before trying any alternative treatments.

Condition	Over-the-Counter Medication with no known harmful effects	Natural Non-Drug Therapies
Allergy	Benadryl Chlor-Trimeton Claritin Zyrtec	
Cold and Flu	Tylenol (acetaminophen)	Saline nasal drops or spray Warm salt/water gargle
Constipation	Citrucil Metamucil Milk of Magnesia	Drink plenty of water Natural food solutions, page 47
First Aid Ointment	Neosporin	
Headache	Tylenol (acetaminophen)	Drink water Head and neck massage Natural food solutions, page 50
Heartburn	Maalox Mylanta Pepcid Tums Zantac	Natural food solutions, page 48
Hemorrhoids	Preparation H Tucks	Witch hazel
Nausea	Meclizine	Sea bands Vitamin B6 100 mg tablet Natural food solutions, page 46
Skin Rash	Hydrocortisone cream or ointment Oatmeal bath (Aveeno)	
Yeast Infection	Monistat Gynelotramin	Natural food solutions, page 53

Chapter 3

Clean Burning Fuel

After reading Chapter One, you know what foods are not safe during pregnancy. As long as you avoid these foods, is it free reign to eat whatever? No, nutrition is more important now than ever. Everything you eat will filter through that tiny growing baby. You need all the nutrients you can get to grow the best baby you can and feel energized and happy while doing it.

Eating Mommy Fabulous style means eating *clean burning fuel*. *Clean burning fuel* is food that provides nutrients that keep you healthy and support your growing baby. *Clean burning fuel* gives you energy and allows you to gain weight during pregnancy without packing on excess body fat. This style of eating improves your metabolism so that postpartum weight loss is much easier.

The Mommy Fabulous style of eating does not focus on counting calories, but I briefly want to explain the calorie requirements of pregnancy by exposing the biggest pregnancy nutrition miscommunication: eating for two. This phrase is extremely misleading; you are not eating for two. You are not even eating for one and a half, not even one and one hundredth of a person. In the first trimester the average woman needs no additional calories, but she needs more nutrients from the calories that she does eat. In the second and third trimester an increase of 300 calories per day is required. That is a calorie equivalent of one piece of whole wheat toast with two tablespoons of peanut butter spread on top. As an exercising pregnant woman, you will probably consume more food (or calories) than a pregnant woman who is not exercising, but if you eat well, you don't have to worry about counting calories. Your body will be able to tell you when it needs nutrients. I am going to teach you how to make food choices so you know what to do with the approximate 2,000 calories you eat now, and how to use your additional 300 calories while you are pregnant. Don't worry; you won't have to count calories. I only explain calorie requirements to illustrate how ridiculous the phrase *eating for two* is.

Next, I should confess that I don't believe in diets. I have never been on one and never plan to. In our culture, the use of the word *diet* is misconstrued. The first definition of the word diet in the dictionary is, "What a person or animal usually eats and drinks; daily fare." The definition of the word diet does not refer to restricted calories or portion control, which are usually the things that come to mind. In my experience as a nutritional counselor, I don't believe that these tactics result in lifelong healthy eating habits for most people. What I do believe in is real food; real food, in contrast to crap. The word *diet* from here forward will only refer to what is eaten, not how much, and in no way will convey the usual connotation of an attempt to lose weight. During pregnancy, the goal is to gain weight in a healthy and controlled manner.

Would you put sugar or garbage in the tank of your sports car? Do you think your car runs very well with sugar or garbage in the tank whether gas is present or not? So why would you fill up on junk and expect your body to function or look its best? How can you expect your body to grow a perfectly healthy baby with crap food as your fuel? My pregnancy (and lifetime) diet is based on a philosophy I call *Cut the Crap*. Whether you are pregnant or not, I see no reason why any person should eat the following twenty-four items, not even in moderation. These items are empty calories, providing no nutritional benefit. If you really can't live without something on this list, limit it to five or six times a year.

Foods containing High Fructose Corn Syrup (HFCS)
Foods that contain trans fat, hydrogenated or partially hydrogenated oils
Foods that have been artificial colored and flavored
Mayonnaise
Gravy
Sour cream
Whipped cream, marshmallows
Canned fruit, vegetables or soup
Caffeine
Mochas, frappuccinos and other blended coffee drinks
Coffee creamers
Soda
Flavored water, sport or energy drinks
White bread products (white bread, plain bagels, sourdough)
Sugar cereal
Scones or muffins or bread with frosting on top
Pastries unless they are from an expensive French bakery
Doughnuts
Fake fruit gel filling in pies or pastries
Fried food
Chips, except unsalted corn chips when eaten with homemade guacamole
Any packaged candy that can be bought at a gas station
Processed or cured meat
Fast food (anything that can be super sized or called a value combo)

Many nutritionists encourage moderation; I am not a supporter for many reasons. My idea of moderation is to have caffeine approximately five times a year. For other people, moderation of caffeine is three times per week. What exactly is moderation? Realistically, most people don't keep track, and who wants to? I feel it is much easier to eat what you want, anytime, and have a list of food that you simply won't touch, much the way a vegetarian doesn't eat steak or someone with a nut allergy doesn't eat peanut butter. Otherwise you will constantly have to evaluate a dish to see if it is a moderate amount of something, or judge how often you should eat it, or whether you can eat that candy bar based on the fact that you already ate a doughnut. Wait… what is being moderated? Doughnuts? Fat? Or sugar? Furthermore, if you eat all twenty-four of these items in *moderation*, aren't you just eating crap all the time in different forms?

I don't feel that these twenty-four items can be considered food. According to the American Heritage® Dictionary the definition of food is: material, usually of plant or animal origin, that contains or consists of essential body nutrients, such as carbohydrates, fats, proteins, vitamins, or minerals, and is ingested and assimilated by an organism to produce energy, stimulate growth, and maintain life. These crap items are devoid of nutrients, vitamins and minerals. In some ways they inhibit growth and shorten the duration and quality of life. Let me explain why these items made the *Cut the Crap* list.

High Fructose Corn Syrup

High fructose corn syrup (HFCS) is a sweetener added to foods. It has been used increasingly in the US over the last 30 years. High fructose corn syrup is extremely soluble and mixes well in many foods. It's inexpensive to make, easy to transport and keeps foods moist. HFCS is so sweet that it is more cost effective for companies to use small quantities of it in place of other, more expensive, sweeteners or flavorings. It is being added to everything from bread to pasta sauces to bacon to beer as well as "health products" like protein bars and "natural" sodas. Studies have shown HFCS can lead to higher caloric intake and therefore can lead to an increase in bodyweight. It fools your body into thinking it's hungry because the body does not recognize or metabolize HFCS as it does natural sugar. When you eat foods with HFCS, you begin to crave HFCS, so it increases the amount of processed foods you eat, thereby decreasing your intake of nutrient-dense foods. Studies are also finding that HFCS may increase insulin resistance and the amount of triglycerides in the bloodstream which could result in increased risk for diabetes.[15] The following foods are usually high in HFCS: soft drinks, fruit drinks and fruit juices that are not 100 % juice, pancake syrups, popsicles, fruit-flavored yogurts, frozen yogurts, ketchup, BBQ sauces, jarred and canned pasta sauces, canned soups, canned fruits (if not in its own juice) and breakfast cereals. Read the ingredients on the label and choose a brand that contains no high fructose corn syrup.

Hydrogenated or Partially Hydrogenated Oils

Avoid foods that contain hydrogenated or partially hydrogenated oils also known as trans fat. The process of hydrogenating oil changes the composition of fat into a form that raises a person's cholesterol when consumed. Hydrogenated or partially hydrogenated oils can be found on a food label under the ingredients list in many processed food products. If you compare labels, you can usually find a different brand of crackers or granola bars that don't contain them. Buyer beware! Manufacturers are sneaky. Trans fat is a new hot topic that consumers are becoming increasingly aware of. In response, manufacturers are now placing "no trans fat" labels on the front of packaging, but if you look at the ingredients you will still find the word hydrogenated oil; avoid these foods. Manufacturers are able to get away with this because lax labeling laws allow small amounts of hydrogenated oils to be labeled as "trans fat-free," which is obviously untrue. Margarine and coffee creamers are common products that contain trans fat. Instead, use real butter sparingly and use non-fat milk and sugar, or chocolate soy milk to flavor your coffee. Trans fats have such a negative effect on cholesterol and overall health that they have been banned in Denmark and Switzerland.[16] If hydrogenated oils are so bad for your health that countries are banning them, why are you still eating them?

Artificial Food Coloring

Prior to World War II, food was colored by using plant extracts. Beets were used to make food pink or red for example. Since then, the chemical industry has developed artificial, chemical coloring derived from petroleum, acetone or coal tars. These are being added to food more frequently because it is cheaper and has infinite shelf life. The problem is that until recently, studies didn't examine how exposure to these chemicals affects humans, their behavior or pregnancy. Even today, many toxicologists feel the FDA and Environmental Protection Agency don't require enough testing of chemicals for subtle effects on neurological processes. The adult brain has a blood brain barrier; it is a protective filter that blocks many chemicals from entering the brain. During the forth week of pregnancy, your baby's brain begins growing. Unlike you, your baby does not have a functional blood brain barrier to protect itself from toxic chemicals. This lack of natural defense allows chemicals into the baby's brain with the potential to cause serious harm and disruption in the brain growth process. An increasing number of chemicals that were not present 30 to 50 years ago are being identified, that can weaken or damage the brain development process. The effects of these chemicals can surface years later as learning disabilities, attention deficit disorder, mental retardation or personality and behavior difficulties such as shyness, hyperactivity and aggression or even violent tendencies and lack of conscience. Researchers have confirmed in a number of studies that children with learning disabilities and attention deficit disorder have at least one of several types of damage to their brain structure.[17] The studies do not point to one specific artificial color, but rather suggest that exposure to a variety of synthetic chemicals can cause problems.[17] While the subject is still controversial, I firmly believe that if it is not natural our bodies can not process it and there will be side effects. Whether you are pregnant or not, artificially colored and flavored foods should be avoided. It is not just the neon pink candy and frosting you need to watch out for; some manufacturers are using artificial colors to dye bread brown so it will look like whole wheat. Examine the ingredienet list of food labels and avoid items containing artificial ingredients such as "FD&C Blue No.1," "Yellow 6" or "artificial flavors," including monosodium glutamate (MSG).

Mayonnaise and Gravy

Mayonnaise and gravy are basically fat, cholesterol and salt. The average person gets enough of these in their daily diet; you don't need to put this crap on top of food. Mayonnaise and gravy mask the taste of any food they cover. Cutting these crap toppings will allow you to taste and enjoy real food. Avoiding mayonnaise means avoiding tartar sauce, hollandaise sauce and Thousand Island dressing which all contain mayonnaise. Mayonnaise provides no real nutritional benefit and is only used to add flavor, or should I say fat, to a dish. Substitute vinegar and olive oil, mustard, chipotle paste or hot sauce to flavor foods and skip the excess salt and fat.

Sour Cream

Sour cream has way too much fat per serving to be consumed and no other redeeming qualities. Fat can be divided into saturated and unsaturated fat. While you generally want to choose foods that are lower in total fat, it is more important to choose foods that contain low to no saturated and trans fat. Your body needs fat to function, and unsaturated fat is best. Your body does not need any saturated or trans fat, so you should aim to consume as little as possible of these two types of fat. Consumption of saturated and trans fats increases your risks for heart disease and raises your cholesterol. You may think that you can still eat fatty foods like sour cream if you choose low fat, reduced fat or light options. I don't care if the label says low or reduced fat. If it is a high fat item like sour cream, then it still contains too much fat. When an item has had the fat reduced, it is usually replaced by sugar or artificial substitutes. Is there a reason you can't eat your vegetables without putting lard on them? Stop using sour cream to avoid the delicious taste of real vegetables and dishes.

Whipped Cream and Marshmallows

Whipped cream and marshmallows are merely sugar and fat, and mostly saturated fat at that. They may also contain high fructose corn syrup, artificial flavors and hydrogenated oils. You may think you can avoid sugar and fat by buying a "light" or "fat free" version; the nutrition label may have a bunch of zeros or ones on them, as if the whipped cream was made of nothing. Don't be fooled. Look to the label where it lists the "percentage of calories from fat." It may list total fat as one gram or less with a 2% Daily Value (sounds good), but the percentage of fat in one serving is 66%. As a general rule you shouldn't eat processed foods with a nutrition label that has more than 30% of the calories coming from fat. Further, the serving size may be only two tablespoons and most people use five tablespoons or more. Be happy eating strawberries, you don't need a dollop of fat on top. Avoid recipes that call for mixing whipped cream with other ingredients. These so called "light" desserts are heavy in calories and light in nutrients.

Canned Foods

Canned foods are kept from rotting on shelves by filling them with salt. Excess dietary salt dehydrates, makes the body retain water and is addictive to the taste buds. Opt for fresh or frozen vegetables instead of canned and make your own soup. Avoid recipes that call for chicken or vegetable stock which contains high amounts of salt and choose recipes that use fresh ingredients. Canned fruit is high in sugar, but not fruit sugar, added refined sugar syrup. Choose fresh fruit or applesauce with "no added sugar." The best applesauce options are the ones with the shortest ingredient list. I do buy canned beans, because I am not going to boil my own kidney beans. There are manufactures that are now offering "no salt added" or "reduced salt" versions. Be sure to check can labels and try to buy brands with sodium at about 12% Daily Value or less.

Caffeine

Caffeine was already discussed with regards to pregnancy in Chapter One. Here I want to explain why it should be omitted from everyone's diet. Caffeine causes difficulty in falling asleep and causes non-restful slumber after you have fallen asleep. The half life of caffeine is six hours, which means that if you drink a caffeinated beverage (100mg caffeine) at nine am, then six hours later, at three pm, there is still 50 mg of caffeine in your system. At bedtime, you still have almost a forth of the caffeine in your system! Caffeine interferes with your ability to get deep sleep. A person who drinks coffee then feels like they need coffee upon waking in the morning. Ditch the caffeine and wake up feeling refreshed! Inadequate sleep is associated with weight gain and inability to lose weight. Caffeine also causes mood swings, fatigue, depression, headaches, stomach upsets and heartburn. If you drink caffeine often, you may have become desensitized to these effects, but you are probably dependant on the stimulant effects and may experience withdrawal symptoms when you reduce caffeine consumption. No one should take addictive substances. Caffeine is often added to diet pills and drinks because of its effect on fat metabolism, but the effect is fleeting. Based on my experience as a trainer and nutritional counselor I recommend not messing with your metabolism with short acting drugs. Exercise to boost your metabolism the healthy way that will have long term benefits.

Flavored Coffee Drinks

When it comes to coffee drinks, I have many issues. I would like to start by saying that I love the taste of coffee, so it is not like I don't drink coffee myself. My first issue is the caffeine. You can, of course, enjoy decaffeinated coffee. My second issue is with the fancy drinks. Carmel macchiato, mint chip frappuccino, peppermint mocha, they all sound lovely, but do you have any idea how many calories, grams of sugar and fat are packed into those? A medium size drink can have 340-470 calories! That is the same number of calories, if not more, in a whole balanced meal! These drinks can have up to 60 grams of sugar! Can I have a little coffee with my sugar? You know the caramel and chocolate syrup contain high fructose corn syrup. My third issue is that there are very few nutrients in these drinks. At least if you get one with milk in it you are getting a little calcium. A person really can't afford to get no nutrients out of 470 calories whether they are pregnant or not. My final issue is with serving sizes. A serving of coffee is 8 oz. Even the smallest size at many places is a 12 oz. to-go cup. If you can't live without take-out coffee, please don't super size your drink or your hips by ordering anything other than a small. When you skip the whipped cream you can cut up to 120 calories. A reasonable coffee drink is a small, non-fat, decaf latte or a small coffee that you add milk and sugar to yourself. Use real sugar and avoid the artificial sweeteners.

Coffee Creamer

You would never (I hope) pour yourself a glass of half and half and drink it. Yet that is often what a coffee creamer is. This is too much fat to add to your coffee. Opt for non-fat milk and natural sugar. Flavored coffee creamers usually contain hydrogenated oils, high fructose corn syrup and artificial flavors.

Soda

Do I need to explain this one? My first issue is the caffeine. If you opt for caffeine free, fine, but I have other issues with soda. Soda contains way too much sugar to be consumed in one beverage. You should consume no more than 50g of sugar a day (World Health Organization recommendation) and one soda can have 46g of sugar. If you opt for a diet or low calorie soda, then the sugar has been substituted for an artificial sweetener. I will discuss sweeteners later in this chapter, but the word artificial should be a red flag. Finally, soda can be high is sodium, which leaves you dehydrated, or at least still thirsty which usually results in additional calorie consumption.

Flavored Water, Sport or Energy Drinks

Flavored water, sport and energy drinks are a source of calories, but not much else. Energy drinks contain excessive amounts of caffeine and other chemicals. Sport drinks are marketed to replace vitamins, minerals and electrolytes lost during exercise. This sort of *replenishment* is only necessary for people training to compete at high levels of competition such as colligate sports, professional or Olympic athletes or for people who do activities like running marathons. There is no significant electrolyte loss unless training is at a high intensity and lasts longer than 60 minutes. While pregnant, it is very unlikely that you will be training this way and it's unlikely you train this way even when you are not pregnant. When you choose flavored water or sport drinks, you are consuming excess calories instead of drinking plain water (zero calories). If you burned 200 calories during the workout and consumed a beverage containing 60 calories, your net is only 140 calories burned. Bummer! During the third trimester, you may only be burning 100 calories during a walk. If you consume one of these pointless drinks, you will be cutting your gains in half, not to mention exposing yourself and your baby to chemicals in the form of artificial colors, favors and sweeteners. If regular water is too boring for you, drop or squeeze a piece of fruit in it.

Sugar Cereals

Sugar cereals are a waste of calories. Sure some of them are fortified with added vitamins, but they do not have the fiber, protein and grains that can be found in other cereals. They usually contain artificial colors and too much refined sugar. Further, starting out your day with sugar cereal will sabotage your food choices all day due to the high glycemic load. The concept of glycemic load will be explained later in this chapter.

White Bread Products

White bread products include sourdough, French bread, plain bagels and buttermilk pancakes. These are a complete waste of calories. First, white bread has been processed by bleaching the color out and therefore destroying the grain. They provide few nutrients for the calories and don't fill you up. You could eat these items and still be hungry later, causing you to overeat without realizing it. Eat whole grains and you will get fiber and protein. You will feel full sooner, and it will take longer for you to feel hungry again. White bread is also high in salt and has a high glycemic load (explained later in the chapter), which can cause cravings. Look for bread that has nuts and seeds in it for added nutrients. Don't be fooled into buying any of this cracked wheat stuff; you are looking for the words: "whole grain" or "whole wheat." Instead of having starchy, bleached out, buttermilk pancakes, look for honey wheat pancake mix and add fresh blueberries; now that's Mommy Fabulous!

Bread that has icing or frosting on top

When you see zucchini bread that has icing or frosting on top it is a big red flag that it's made with too much refined sugar, fat and other cheap ingredients. There is nothing wrong with muffins, scones or other bread products which can be made with whole grains and contain fruits, vegetables, seeds or nuts. Your best bet is to make these yourself so you can see how much sugar and butter are in them, I always use half the sugar a recipe calls for and never miss it.

Pastries

Pastries include coffee cakes, Danishes, éclairs and cinnamon buns. Obviously these items are not a source of nutrients or vitamins. Usually these are made of refined sugar, HFCS, bleached flour, artificial flavors and colors and saturated fat. So why do I condone these items when purchased from an expensive European bakery? Well, you do have to enjoy life a little. A pastry from an expensive privately owned bakery (no chain bakeries) is usually made with top of the line ingredients and usually with real natural flavors. They are still fatty and not healthy, but at least they are not complete junk. So enjoy… it is not everyday that you come across an expensive French bakery or can afford a $4 croissant topped with toasted almonds and filled with all natural raspberry preserves. But please, don't ever eat a pastry from a plastic package or from a gas station!!!!!! Real food rots, so anything with a long shelf life contains chemicals.

Doughnuts

A doughnut is made of saturated fat, trans fat, bleached flour and then fried in fat and frosted with artificially colored and sweetened frosting. If that weren't bad enough they are sometimes injected with gelatinous fake fruit gel or disgusting pudding. I don't think doughnuts can be considered food. Indulge in something delicious like a pie made with real apples. Please don't abuse your body by eating a crappy doughnut. Did I mention that a doughnut has between 200 to 380 calories and a high glycemic load?

Fake fruit gel filling in pies or pastries

I recommend eating a real fruit filled pie as a smart dessert choice. But if you don't make it yourself, you will often find that a pie is filled with gel filling, artificially dyed the color of a fruit. You may find a few pieces of fruit saturated with refined sugar floating in this gelatinous muck. Why would you eat this? It sounds disguising because it is disgusting. Find a baker who sells real fruit pies, or make one yourself. Use ¼ to ½ of the sugar a recipe calls for and extra cinnamon or nutmeg. The pie will still taste delicious and you will be getting more nutrients per calorie consumed without exposing yourself or your baby to chemical additives.

Any Fried Foods

Don't even try to pass off turkey bacon as a health food. It may have less saturated fat than pig bacon, but you still fry it. I have even had people tell me that they don't fry it; they put it in the microwave. The fat content warms up and it fries...hello! People falsely believe that frying at home is a health decision. Something that is not *as bad* for you is not the same as something that is good for you. Even using vegetable oil instead of lard so that the frying isn't "that bad" doesn't cut it. Natural fatty acids in oil are converted to carcinogenic (cancer-causing) substances at frying temperatures. Tempura doesn't pass either. Frying vegetables destroys their health benefits.

Chips

Chips often contain artificial colors and flavors and are usually high in salt, not to mention they have low to no protein, fiber, vitamins or minerals. They also have a high glycemic load, explained later in the chapter. Ironically, corn and potatoes are quite healthy vegetables. The process of converting them into chip form obliterates the vegetable, converting it into something that is no longer real food, but food-like. Corn and potatoes don't come in other flavors, so neither should chips. Any cereal-pretzel mix like Chex-Mix falls into the chip category because of their similarly unhealthy ingredients. Homemade guacamole made of smashed avocado mixed with an all natural salsa containing corn kernels, black beans and tomatoes is incredibly healthy and who is going to eat that with a spoon? Compare labels and find the healthiest all natural corn chip you can with no added salt. Chips with no added salt usually advertise that right on the front of the bag, so they are easy to spot. You should eat more guacamole than chips; the chip should serve as an edible spoon.

Packaged Candy

Packaged candy is at the bottom of the food quality list, and also at the bottom of the candy quality list. Packaged candy is highly processed, contains artificial flavors, colors, high fructose corn syrup, trans fat, saturated fat and has a high glycemic load. Most granola bars covered in chocolate or made with chocolate chips are also candy bars, try not to kid yourself. Because packaged candy is so convenient at grocery stores, gas stations and vending machines, people have gotten the impression that it is a snack. Candy is not a snack! As a rule, never eat candy when you are hungry. If you want to eat candy, it should be after you have eaten a meal. When you make a candy selection, it should not be artificially colored or contain anything from the *Cut the Crap* list. If you are interested in nature's candy, there is nothing sweeter than a Medjool date. They are so deliciously sweet when they are not pitted. A box of raisins or an all natural granola bar made with honey could also satisfy your sweet tooth. Pop Quiz: If it is a holiday and there is a box of candy purchased from a chocolatier, which chocolate do you choose to eat: the caramel-marshmallow, the jelly filled cherry chocolate or the chocolate covered nut cluster? Have you learned anything...the nut cluster, of course! At the very least you are getting some protein out of it, there is nothing redeemable about the other options.

Processed Meats

Processed meats include jerky, bologna, sausage, bacon, hot dogs, corned beef, pepperoni, chicken nuggets, fish sticks and other such oddities. They are usually fatty, salty, void of nutrients and high in preservatives. Often the left over junk after butchering is complete is what is used to produce these processed meats. For example, after the chicken is butchered into thighs, breasts and drumsticks, whatever is leftover on the carcass is scrapped off and put into a machine that smashes it into a nugget. It is then deep fried so you don't realize it's the scraps you wouldn't eat. In order to sell a poor quality meat, a manufacturer can *cure* it. This is done by heavily salting meat and leaving it to sit until it is completely dehydrated, viola, jerky! If you can't identify what part of the animal the item comes from you should pass on it. Where are the nuggets on a chicken, the bacon on a pig or the sausage of a cow? One of the preservatives used to extend the shelf life of processed meat is sodium nitrate. Sodium nitrate is suspected of increasing cancer risk and The Center for Science in the Public Interest recommends limiting the amount you consume. Processing renders food less healthy and in some cases dangerous. It is the processing procedure that resulted in the contamination of ground beef with the infectious agent that causes Mad Cow Disease in humans. There are many other epidemiologic studies that suggest the ways foods are processed cause illnesses. Do yourself a favor and choose real cuts of meat.

Fast Food

There are certain items on the menu at fast food chains that can be healthy, but when it comes to fast food, I believe in guilt by association. Any of these supposedly *healthy* food choices spend the day around deep fryers, grease and processed foods. I feel that the marketing can be misleading as to the real nutritional value of these food items. *Lite* menu items may have less fat than other menu items, but may still be fattier than lunch you would get elsewhere. *Balanced* fast food meals may serve apple slices or lettuce with fried chicken, but I am a little confused on how a few apple slices *balance* a fried chicken. You are still eating crap (fried chicken) even if it is next to something that is not crap. The phrase *value menu* is a red flag. Value menu means more saturated fat per dollar spent. Who wants more fat per dollar? In fact, the best quality food usually means you get less fat per dollar spent...it is a trick! Super sized is also a red flag. If you will notice, only crap can be super sized: soda, fries, slushies. There is already too much fat, sugar, caffeine and cholesterol in the item as it is and then you want to super size it? I would like to see a fast food restaurant super size an orange or a carrot. Always order the smallest size, whether it is a coffee drink, a smoothie or a hamburger. Today's sizes (and super sizes) are so big they are actually two to three servings. The smallest size is already too much. There should be no question as to whether anyone needs a medium or large. It is best to avoid fast food menus. If it is late at night, everything is closed and you have nothing at home because you didn't get a chance to go grocery shopping, then try to pick the healthiest thing on the menu. Most of the time fast food is consumed as a result of poor planning and a lack of commitment to your health. If you plan ahead, you will have snacks on hand to tide you over until you can get some real food. The grocery store is easy too. Get out of the car and get yourself some ready-made food such as a sandwich or a salad instead of a value combo.

Reduce this Crap

Salt (Sodium)
Sugar

Salt and sugar are flavoring disasters. When they occur naturally in foods they are healthy. When they are added to dishes, they mask the actual taste of real food and are addictive to the taste buds. You may crave the salt, not the actual food you are putting the salt on. If you keep a salt shaker on the table, throw it away! Excess salt in the diet increases the risk of high blood pressure for everyone. Pregnant women are very sensitive to high blood pressure because they already have a higher blood volume than before. In addition, excess salt intake can lead to swelling. Many pregnant women experience some swelling, especially of the feet at the end of the day. Add some salty foods like chips, canned foods or soy sauce (all crap) and you won't be able to fit in your shoes. A client came to me stating that she thought she was eating a healthy diet, not realizing it was high in salt. Her swelling was so bad she had to wear sandals in the winter until she reduced her salt intake and the swelling subsided. Here are some easy ways to cut salt out of the diet. Stop salting the pasta cooking water. Add salt according to the recipe while cooking, not on top after. If a recipe says salt is optional, leave it out. Season food with garlic, chopped chives, lemon juice, olive oil, vinegar, pepper or other dry spices and you won't notice a lack of salt. Cut high salt foods like canned soups or vegetables, gravy, lunch meats, pickles, white bread products and all processed foods. Stop making food that comes out of a box, which is usually high in sodium. Try not to buy anything that contains more than 200 mg of sodium per serving. If you are going to buy a box mix like rice pilaf compare the labels and buy the brand that is lower in sodium.

Added sugar also masks real food flavor. Many people don't realize just how much refined sugar they are consuming during the day. To discuss sugar, we must divide it into two categories: simple sugars, which you want to minimize consumption of, and complex carbohydrates which you will not have to moderate if you make wise food choices. There is one caveat to minimizing simple sugar intake. Technically fruit contains simple sugar, but you should NOT reduce fruit consumption. No one ever got fat from eating fruit (it was the other crap they ate) and no pregnant woman gained thirty pounds in her first trimester because she ate tons of cantaloupe. Fruit contains lots of nutrients, fiber and water.

Excess consumption of sugar and calories can result in unnecessary weight gain which increases the risk of developing Type II diabetes or for the pregnant woman, gestational diabetes. Healthy women with no family history can develop gestational diabetes. When a pregnant woman develops gestational diabetes it may go away after she delivers, but she now has up to a 50% chance of developing Type II diabetes within ten years. Even if you have diabetes prone genetics, the disease can be prevented, managed and even treated with proper nutrition and exercise. Another reason to limit simple sugar intake during pregnancy is that you are more vulnerable to developing cavities. This may result from hormonal changes or because pregnant women tend to eat more times a day, exposing their teeth to more sugar.

Check the chart below to see what simple sugar foods should be cut and which complex carbohydrate foods can be eaten to your heart's content. I hope you stop ruining perfectly good food (fruit and cereal) by sprinkling processed, refined sugar on it.

Avoid Simple Sugars	Enjoy Complex Carbohydrates
Soda, flavored water, fruit drinks	Real fruit smoothie made with milk or yogurt
Mocha	Smoothie: Decaf coffee, milk, ice, banana
Sugar cereal	Oatmeal, bran flakes, shredded wheat
White bread	Whole wheat bread
Pretzels, chips	Whole wheat crackers, plain popcorn
Doughnuts, pastries	Bran muffins, whole wheat bagel
Candy	Granola bars containing oats and nuts
Buttermilk pancakes	Oat bran, buckwheat or honey wheat pancakes
White baking flour (bleached)	Substitute half with whole wheat flour in recipes

Whole grains are awesome!

Studies have shown that people who consume more whole grains generally have better weight management.[18] Whole grains have been shown to reduce the risk of cardiovascular disease, diabetes, and high blood pressure.[18] They also reduce the risk of developing cancer.[18] You may be eating fewer whole grains than you think because food labeling can be deceiving. The words bran, multi-grain, stone-ground, 100% wheat or cracked wheat is usually NOT whole grain. Look at the ingredients list; "whole grain" should be the first or second ingredient.

When you first cut back on salt and sugar foods may taste bland. It takes about a month to break the salt-sugar addiction. Once the addiction is broken, you will begin to enjoy the actual flavor of foods. If you are currently eating crap, you will be surprised at the many different flavors and dishes you will come to enjoy when you are free from processed flavors and can actually taste real food. Foods you once thought were bland will begin to taste interesting. You may find that Indian food, curry or Italian dishes are a lot tastier than you previously thought. Fruit will begin to taste very sweet. After living your new diet, you will find that when you are offered cake at a birthday party, you will not be interested in finishing it. It will taste too sweet, or be too rich or it will taste like cheap imitation food because your taste buds will be used to the taste and texture of real food.

Cutting crap from your diet may sound like a diet in the restrictive sense of the word, but it is actually quite liberating. Once you *Cut the Crap*, you are free to eat anything you want without having to worry about moderation, calories, portion sizes or guilt. While you are pregnant your body needs so many nutrients that you really don't have calories to spare on junk. *Cut the Crap* and you can use those calories to eat something that will fuel you and your baby without over-consuming total calories and gaining excessive weight. Finally you should notice that you are more energized, have fewer cravings and are less moody with these foods out of your life. This lifestyle should not feel restrictive. Now that you know these items are crap, and you break the addiction, you won't want any of them. This lifestyle is something you maintain the rest of your life whether pregnant or not, and it is something you should follow when feeding your children. Maybe I should change the name from *Cut the Crap* to Free-to-be-Fabulous.

Glycemic Load
how the concept can help you stay fit

The goal during pregnancy is to gain weight, so I don't believe you should focus on calories. I don't think it is the best strategy for anyone to eat healthy; it's more important to make wise food choices. Glycemic load is a concept that can help you make these choices. A food with a high glycemic load will cause your blood sugar to rise quickly after consumption. Foods with a low glycemic load break down more slowly and moderately increase blood sugar levels over time. When you eat foods with a high glycemic load, they often don't fill you up and they cause you to crave more sugar or salt. This increase in appetite will lead you to eat more food than you need to and therefore gain more weight than you need to. Additionally, after a food with a high glycemic load gives you a sugar rush, it will then be followed by a blood sugar drop. For the pregnant woman, this can cause lightheadedness, feeling fatigue and craving more sugar. Smart food choices will help you maintain stable blood sugar, keep cravings to a minimum and prevent energy crashes. There is a connection between what you eat and whether or not you will have enough energy to go to the gym. Don't underestimate it.

As a general rule, the more processed a food the higher the glycemic load. Most items on the *Cut the Crap* list have a high glycemic load. Real food can also have a high glycemic load. For example, mashed potatoes have a higher glycemic load than a whole baked potato. Potatoes processed into chips have an even higher glycemic load. Glycemic load, or blood sugar effect, does not necessarily equate with the amount of sugar in an item, it has more to do with the extent an item is processed. For example, most fruit has a low glycemic load, whereas fruit juice has a much greater impact on your blood sugar. Fruit syrup would have an even larger impact on blood sugar.

When you eat food with a high glycemic load, you can consume it with other low glycemic load foods to balance out the overall effect on blood sugar levels. Fat and fiber tend to lower the glycemic effect when eaten with foods. If you are going to eat buttermilk pancakes and juice (both have a high glycemic load) for breakfast you will experience a blood sugar spike and a blood sugar drop. Instead, balance a glass of juice with whole wheat toast and a hard boiled egg to keep blood sugar steady longer. The best food strategy for keeping your blood sugar level, cravings at bay and maintain energy is to not eat bread products alone. Eat corn chips with guacamole, crackers with cheese and spaghetti with meatballs. The following chapters will give you food suggestions and recipes that will help you to recognize balanced and tasty combinations.

There are a lot of funny pregnancy craving stories, but if you maintain steady blood sugar levels, cravings will be minimal. I craved fruit during my first trimester (which has a low glycemic load), but after that I really had no cravings for any specific food. It is a myth that a food craving is based on a biological need. A pregnant woman who craves pickles probably doesn't need salt. She craves salt because she is probably eating too much salt, so her taste buds are accustomed to salty foods and respond positively to that taste. It is important to manage cravings because it can be the difference between gaining the perfect amount of weight and gaining excessive weight in a short amount of time.

Glycemic Load Chart

Compare the foods and choose to eat those with a lower glycemic load.

Food	Serving Size	Glycemic Load
Strawberries	1 cup	Very Low
Strawberry pop tart	1 pop tart	High
Popcorn	3 cups	Low
Graham cracker	1 cracker	High
Low fat fruit flavored yogurt	½ cup	Low
Bagel	1 medium size	Very High
Tortilla, corn or wheat	1 medium size	Low
Hamburger bun, white	Top and bottom	Very High
Ice cream, vanilla	1 cup	Low
Low fat ice cream, vanilla	1 cup	High
Peanuts	½ cup	Insignificant
Pretzels	1 oz.	High
Pizza	1 large slice	Low
Macaroni & cheese	1 cup	Very High

Can I substitute?

Consuming sugar causes your blood sugar level to rise sharply and then plummet. Sugar consumption can also lead to cavities. Sugar is natural, but its not perfect. There are many sugar substitutes on the market claiming to be a better choice than sugar. They are getting a lot of attention and stirring up controversy. There are currently five Food and Drug Administration (FDA) approved artificial sweeteners: saccharin (Sweet'N Low), aspartame (NutraSweet, Equal), acesulfame potassium (Sunett), sucralose (Splenda), and neotame.

Saccharin (Sweet 'N Low) crosses the placenta so it should be avoided during pregnancy. Some scientists believe that infant formula containing saccharin causes irritability and muscle dysfunction in infants.

Aspartame (NutraSweet, Equal) is one of the most controversial nutrition topics. Nothing has been definitively proven, but aspartame is being linked with cancers, chronic diseases, increased hunger, nausea and more.[19] Without conclusive evidence, the FDA will not issue warnings, so it is currently labeled as safe during pregnancy and lactation.

Neotame is a newer version of aspartame and is also labeled as safe during pregnancy and lactation by the FDA.

Acesulfame potassium (Sunett) contains a cancer causing agent called methylene chloride. Long-term exposure to methylene chloride can cause headaches, depression, nausea, mental confusion, liver effects, kidney effects, visual disturbances, and cancer in humans. There has been a great deal of opposition to the use of acesulfame K without further testing, but at this time, the FDA has not required that these tests be done so it continues to be labeled as safe during pregnancy and lactation. [19]

Sucralose (Splenda) is controversial because it was discovered by scientists while trying to create a new insecticide. The Splenda website states, "…although sucralose has a structure like sugar and a sugar-like taste, it is not natural." The presence of chlorine is thought to be the most dangerous component of sucralose. Chlorine is considered a carcinogen and has been used in poisonous gas, disinfectants, pesticides, and plastics. The alleged symptoms associated with sucralose are chest pains, diarrhea, gas and nausea, allergic reactions including rash, hives, itchy eyes, swelling, wheezing, cough, runny nose, and physiological problems including anxiety, anger, moods swings and depression. The only way to be sure of the safety of sucralose is to conduct long-term studies on humans. Sucralose has no calories, has no effect on blood sugar (no glycemic load), and is labeled safe during pregnancy and lactation.

You may be able to tell that I am biased against artificial sweeteners. The FDA has reviewed research on these artificial sweeteners and has deemed them safe for consumption during pregnancy, with the exception of saccharin. There are many research groups that are finding links between artificial sweetener consumption and various forms of cancer in animals.[19] I do not recommend artificial sweeteners (for anyone) because of the lack of long term studies to support their safety. Unfortunately, this is a situation where artificial flavors must be proven harmful to the FDA rather than having to be proven safe before consumption. Why eat something until it is actually proven safe, especially while pregnant? The American Pregnancy Association recommends that women with diabetes or gestational diabetes should limit their exposure to sweeteners. Isn't the word artificial a red flag? Why would a fabulous person like you eat something that is artificial?

Is a diet soda better than a regular one?

With regards to soda, *diet* usually means sugar has been replaced with no calorie artificial sweeteners. A diet soda generally has the same nutrition label as a regular soda with fewer calories. Perhaps, diet soda is a better choice. Am I proud of the decision? No. Soda has no nutritional value; it's crap. The mere existence of artificial sweeteners makes you think you are making smart choices, when you should be choosing foods that don't come in *diet*.

In a study where researchers fed rats a food sweetened with a no calorie sweetener (that is, a food that was actually lower in total calories) the rats ate more food and gained more weight than rats given food with real sugar that was higher in total calories. If overeating wasn't bad enough, rats eating the no-calorie sweetened food adjusted their body's metabolic processes to burn fewer calories contributing to increased bodyweight and fat.[20]

Sugar Alcohols

There is an alternative to sugar and artificial sweeteners. Sugar alcohols are often found in foods labeled as "sugar free." Sugar alcohols are not sugar, but rather carbohydrates. Examples of sugar alcohols include sorbitol, erthritol, xylitol, isomalt, mannitol and Hydrogenated Starch. Stevia, Truvia and PureVia are a few of the brands you may recognize. Sugar alcohols occur naturally in plants. Some of them are extracted from plants (sorbitol from corn syrup, mannitol from seaweed and erthritol from stevia leaves), but they are mostly manufactured. The impact of sugar alcohols on blood sugar is less than the effect of sugar; in some cases there is no effect on blood sugar. Sugar alcohols provide few to no calories per gram. The reason for this is because they are not completely absorbed in the intestine. Another plus is that sugar alcohols don't promote tooth decay as sugar does.

It seems there are many positives for sugar alcohols, but there may be some drawbacks. First, sugar alcohols are often used in combination with artificial sweeteners. Second, when there is *no sugar* in a cake, people often eat more than they would if it had sugar. It's like people interpret sugar free to mean calorie free. In the end, they may get the same blood sugar response and sometimes even more calories. Another downside is that because sugar alcohols are not completely absorbed, they can ferment in the intestines and cause bloating, gas, or diarrhea. People can have different reactions to different sugar alcohols or no reaction at all. If the product is labeled "sugar-free" or "no added sugar", the manufacturer must show the sugar alcohol count separately on the label. In the end, sugar and sugar alcohols are both empty calories, and both mask the taste of real strawberries. Try to not overindulge your sweet tooth.

For Your Baby

Have a positive relationship with food. You should not read this chapter thinking that it is a drag to eat healthy. You should not think of the *Cut the Crap* list as a list of restrictions, you should think of it as a list of things you don't want to put in your body. You are not denying yourself junk food; you are protecting yourself from inferior products that lead to poor nutrition and disease. You do it because you are worth it.

Your relationship with food will affect your child during pregnancy and after. You can help develop your baby's preferences for food while you are pregnant. It may seem odd, but the flavors of what you eat reach the amniotic fluid, not just the nutrient break down. When you eat spaghetti, think about your baby marinating in a tomato sauce. Studies have shown that babies are born with a predilection for the flavors their mother ate while pregnant.[21] For example, if you eat a lot of marinara sauce, your baby will probably like tomatoes, garlic and oregano. If you eat a lot of curry, your baby may enjoy spicy foods. Food flavors also enter breast milk; another reason to eat healthy. Do you want your baby born with a taste for saturated fat and high fructose corn syrup?

Your job as a parent is to teach your children good eating habits (in addition to everything else) and protect them from poor nutrition (and everything else). Develop a positive relationship with food if you have not already. Food is not for making you feel better, it is not a reward, it should not be used as a punishment and it is not something to do when you are bored. Do not use food this way with yourself, and do not use food to get your children to cooperate with you. Food is for sustaining life, so choose food that has a positive affect on your body and be happy with it.

You may or may not know whether you are having a boy or a girl, but keep this in mind. A mother who has a negative relationship with food and weight is more likely to have a daughter that grows up to have an eating disorder. Of adolescences that do not develop diagnosable eating disorders, twenty percent have unhealthy dieting behaviors aimed at weight loss.[22]

What is served and eaten in your home while your child is young will set the course for how he or she eats for the rest of their life. There is an escalating epidemic of childhood obesity which translates into higher risk for many chronic diseases as they mature into adults. The prevalence of overweight children has doubled since 1980.[23] While food may not be the only factor; most parents don't realize how the foods they are serving their kids are causing health problems. Many of us remember eating macaroni and cheese, hot dogs and cupcakes as kids and we turned out fine, right? What most of us don't understand is that these foods have become far worse over the last twenty years. Many chemical additives didn't exist when we were kids. There wasn't hydrogenated oil in your mac and cheese; there wasn't high fructose corn syrup in your cupcake frosting. Kids today are being exposed to much more processed and chemically altered food than when we were little. So wake up! Don't poison your child's metabolism with crap. Eat healthy while you are pregnant and continue a life of good nutrition after you deliver.

When I knew I had done good

When Talia was twenty months old I bought her a new plate. It was a cute little cafeteria tray with four wells. I was excited to give her the gift and said, "Look Talia, it is a new plate for you." Talia took the plate into her tiny chubby hand and pointed at the first well and said, "Carrots," then pointed to the next and said, "Pasta" (which she pronounced, "Fasta"). Pointing to the third, she said, "Grapes," and then pointed to the last well and said, "Cheese." It was funny she was placing an order, and of course I was proud that she wasn't asking for mac n' cheese, cookies, Cheetos and bologna, but I was shocked and amazed that she had assembled a perfectly balanced meal with all the food groups!

Chapter 4

Eating Fabulously

The Basics

Your meals should include the five basic food groups. Each day you should get the following:

6-11 servings of grains
3-5 servings of vegetables
2-4 servings of fruits
2-3 servings of dairy
2-3 servings of protein (5-7 ounces)

Foods low in fat and high in fiber are important to a healthy diet.

What is with the range? There is a big difference between six and eleven servings of grains.

The United States nutritional recommendations base the number of servings you need on your age, sex, and level of activity.[24] You should follow the grey box below, as I hope you are an active, pregnant woman. There is no need to adjust servings during pregnancy unless you are carrying multiple babies. If so, your needs will be different and you should consult your doctor. During pregnancy you need about ½ ounce more protein for a total of 60-75g a day. You will also need more vitamins and minerals which should be obtained by eating an extra serving of fruit and veggies during the third trimester.

Children 2 to 6, inactive women, some older adults (based on 1,600 calories/day)	Older children, teen girls, active women, most men (based on 2,200 calories/day)	Teen boys, active men (based on 2,800 calories/day)
Milk -- 2 servings Protein -- 5 ounces Vegetable -- 3 servings Fruit -- 2 servings Grains -- 6 servings	Milk -- 2 servings Protein -- 6 ounces Vegetable -- 4 servings Fruit -- 3 servings Grains -- 9 servings	Milk -- 2 servings Protein -- 7 ounces Vegetable -- 5 servings Fruit -- 4 servings Grains -- 11 servings

What does a serving size consist of?

Grain Products: 1 slice of whole wheat bread, ½ whole wheat bagel or bun, 1 cup of dry cereal, ½ cup of cooked cereal like oatmeal, ½ cup of brown rice, ½ cup of whole wheat pasta, 1 small roll or muffin, 2 large multi-grain crackers (refined carbohydrates don't count toward grains)
Vegetables: ½ cup of raw or cooked vegetables, ¾ cup of vegetable juice, 1 cup of raw leafy vegetables
Fruits: 1 medium fruit such as an apple, banana or orange, 1 melon wedge, ½ large fruit such as a grapefruit, ½ cup of berries, ¾ cup of 100% fruit juice, ¼ cup of dried fruit
Dairy: 1 cup of milk, 1 cup of yogurt, 1½ oz. of cheese

Protein: 1 egg, ½ cup of cooked or canned beans, 6 tablespoons of peanut butter, 2 to 3 oz. of lean meat such as fish, skinless poultry or low fat cuts of beef. Three ounces of meat is about the size of a deck of cards. Six Tablespoons of peanut butter is the equivalent of three golf balls.

I am never going to measure my food, does eating healthy have to be that technical?

Most Americans are over consuming carbohydrates and protein and aren't eating the recommended number of servings of fiber and produce they need for good health. So please measure if you want, but I have no time for this either. I have never measured out a serving of anything before sitting down to eat. I just estimate by asking myself a few questions:

Have I eaten two card decks worth of food from the protein group?
Have I eaten three whole fruits or three handfuls of denser fruit (berries, dried fruit, juice)?
Have I eaten two baseballs worth of vegetables?
Have I only eaten whole grains today? There is so much bleached flour in the world that by simply trying to not eat anything that is not whole grain you will probably not surpass six servings. People tend to over-eat bread products, and still not get the grains they need. It is not a bad idea to measure out a serving of cereal once, just so you can see how it looks in a bowl.

How often should I eat while pregnant?

While pregnant, I recommend eating three meals a day and two snacks. Eat breakfast, lunch and dinner at reasonable, consistent times every day. Then have a snack at 10:00 am and again at 3:00 pm. If you are hungry more often than this, add an additional light snack. Try to eat at consistent times, even if you are not hungry. This is the best way to keep your blood sugar steady. When your blood sugar drops it causes you to feel tired, cranky and craving sugar or salt. Remember, steady blood sugar means minimal cravings resulting in energy to workout, healthy weight gain, a strong metabolism, easier postpartum recovery and general happiness all around.

Can I see a sample menu?

Breakfast: banana, low-fat yogurt or oatmeal, decaf coffee with fat-free milk and sugar
Snack: unsalted nuts and a tangerine with water
Lunch: grilled chicken sandwich with provolone cheese and tomato on a whole wheat roll, spinach salad with cranberries and walnuts with an Italian dressing or a vinaigrette and water with lemon
Snack: chocolate soy milk, peanut butter, baby carrots
Dinner: pasta with roasted veggies, salad with chopped cucumber and tomato and water

Many people tend to over-eat pasta, so remember that one cup of pasta is two servings. When you prepare pasta dishes there should almost be as many vegetables as noodles volume-wise, so that every bite is half pasta half veggies.

Snacks
A Mommy's Best Friend

Keep a snack on yourself at all times, just in case. Poor food choices are usually made due to lack of planning. If you are going to be out all morning, you should have your 10:00 am snack with you, plus a back-up. If you think, *oh, I'll just get something at the mall*, then you should plan what it is that you will get at the mall before you get there, and plan to be by that vendor around 10:00 am. Many people who do half-ass planning end up being starved with nothing but a Cinnabon in sight. By making the poor choice to eat *whatever*, they have blown their daily consumption of fat, saturated fat, trans fat, cholesterol, calories, nutrient needs and they have just eaten something with a high glycemic load which will result in a blood sugar spike followed by a drop which can cause undesirable effects on mood and energy. Don't con yourself into thinking this is a *treat*, the reality is that you are sabotaging yourself.

My Favorite Snacks

> Hummus and whole wheat crackers with cheese slices (Piave, Gruyère, Fontina, Smoked Gouda are my favorites)
> Trail mix (nuts, coconut, dried fruit) Find a tropical mix. Dried papaya…yes please!
> Peanut butter and baby carrots, celery sticks or apple slices
> Smoothie or frozen fruit bars or freeze yogurt and berries in a popsicle mold
> Homemade guacamole and unsalted corn chips
> Yogurt parfait (low fat yogurt, granola or cereal, berries)
> Low fat cottage cheese with green apple cubes
> Unsalted nuts or soy nuts and unsweetened applesauce
> Almonds and dried cherries
> Pistachios and dried cranberries
> Grapes with Havarti cheese and whole wheat baguette
> Hard boiled egg white
> Chocolate soy milk
> 5 layer dip with unsalted corn chips-olives, avocado, tomato, cheddar cheese and black or pinto beans (whole beans)

These are some of my favorite snacks because they taste great and most of these snack ideas include multiple food groups, so you are maximizing the amount of nutrients you are getting. A piece of fruit seems like a good snack idea, but it's a better snack strategy to eat fruit with something else. Fruit metabolizes too quickly. You need protein or fat to stave off hunger and tide you over until your next meal. Remember that you may only need an additional 300 calories in the third trimester compared to before you got pregnant, but you need a lot more nutrients. Adding one or two of these snacks per day could be the only calorie addition you need to make while pregnant. Smart snacking is eating for two.

Snack Tip

Keep a bowl of some munchies on the counter. Often when pregnant you could graze and be satisfied with only a few bites to keep your blood sugar level until the next meal. Good counter snacks are a bowl of nuts, trail mix (no chocolate) or grapes. By placing nuts on the counter, you can still gauge how much you are consuming. When the bowl is half empty at the end of the day, you know you grazed one serving of protein. People who graze from packages and cupboards tend to overeat because they don't realize how much was in the box before, or how much is in there afterward and they forget about some of those little nibbles during the day. Cupboard grazers also tend to miscalculate how many food group servings they had. A cupboard grazer who had dried fruit, crackers and nuts many think they had 1 serving of fruit, 1 serving of grains and 1 serving of protein, when they actually only had ½ serving of fruit, 3 servings of carbohydrates and a half serving of protein.

On-the-Go Snacks

All- natural granola bars and fruit leather are great snacks that can be kept in your car or purse. Choose those with the shortest ingredient list. A baggie of unsalted nuts, sunflower seeds or dry cereal can be kept in your car or purse for a long time. Don't buy those terrible prepared party mixes filled with salt and weird flavorings. If you are packing a snack for the day, olives, cherry or grape tomatoes, baby carrots and celery are vegetables that can handle a bumpy ride in a purse and keep pretty well outside a refrigerator. Apples or dried fruit including a box of raisins can handle a purse or backpack. Choose dried fruit with no added sugar. Those with added sugar have additional non- nutrient calories you don't need, and the sugar crystallizes into a crunchiness which is just gross. A single serving unsweetened applesauce container is also a mobile snack. Trail mix is an excellent snack because the nutrients are healthy and from many sources like nuts, seeds and fruit. Skip flavored mixes, where the taste of the real food is masked by sugar, salt and artificial flavors. Likewise, skip mixes with chocolate or yogurt covered contents.

Snack Tip

There may be times when you wake up in the night to use the bathroom and realize that you are starving. Keep grapes in the house. It is very easy to grab a few grapes from a bowl on the counter and go back to bed. If you turn on lights, open the fridge and start moving things around you are just going to fully wake yourself up and binge on something that is probably not the best thing to sit in your stomach the rest of the night. It will also be harder to fall back asleep, and you need your rest!

All Foods Are Not Created Equal

All foods are not created equal, and the food label is where an item reveals its true colors. The very first thing you should look at when examining a food label is the ingredient list. When looking at an ingredient list, like the one below, first look for any of the ingredients that I have bolded. If any of these appear on the label, you should not buy, or eat it. The item is processed crap. Look for a brand that is real food. If the item is a cereal or bread product, the healthiest choices will have "whole wheat flour" as the first or second ingredient.

INGREDIENTS: ENRICHED FLOUR BLEACHED (WHEAT FLOUR NIACIN, IURON, THIAMIN, FOLIC ACID) SUGAR, PARTCIALLY **HYDROGENATED** SOYBEAN OIL, COACO, **HIGH FRUCTOSE CORN SYRUP**, CORN STARCH, PROPYLENE GLYCOL MONOESTERS OF FATTY ACIDS, SALT, DISTILLED MONOGLYCERIDES, **ARTICIACIAL FLAVORS**, CELLULOSE GUM, NONFAT MILK, **YELLOW 6**.

It is pretty simple to scan the ingredients for four items. Also check for **sucralose, acesulfame potassium, aspartame** and **saccharin**, which are all artificial sweeteners. If the item passes the crap ingredient check then I would examine the nutrition facts. Here is what you should look for:

Nutrition Facts	
Serving Size 4 oz. (113g)	
Servings per Container: 4	
Amount per Serving	
Calories 280	Calories from Fat 130
	% Daily Value*
Total Fat 14g	22%
Saturated Fat 3.5g	18%
Trans Fat 2.5 g	
Cholesterol 120mg	40%
Sodium 640mg	27%
Total Carbohydrates 13g	4%
Dietary Fiber 1g	4%
Sugars 0g	
Protein 4g	
Vitamin A 2%	Vitamin C 4%
Calcium 3%	Iron 6%

*Percent Daily Values are based on a 2,000 calorie diet. Your daily values may be higher or lower depending on your calorie needs.

	Calories	2,000	2,500
Total Fat	Less Than	65g	80g
Saturated Fat	Less Than	20g	25g
Cholesterol	Less Than	300mg	300mg
Sodium	Less Than	2400mg	2400mg
Total Carbohydrates		300g	375g
Dietary Fiber		25g	30g
Calories per gram:			
Fat 9	Carbohydrate 4		Protein 4

1. Don't eat anything with Trans Fat in it. If the ingredients don't list a hydrogenated oil then the Trans Fat will be zero.

2. Quickly look down the % Daily Value list. If anything has 20% or more of the Daily Value, besides fiber, then the item is out. In fact, I always feel like 18% is getting too close to 20%. Here we can see that Fat, Saturated Fat, Cholesterol and Sodium are all too high. This item is crap!

3. If the item passes the % Daily Value check, then I would look at carbohydrates. As long as the item does not appear on the *Cut the Crap* list I am not too concerned about how many total carbohydrates it contains. What I am concerned with is the ratio of carbohydrates to sugars. Here there are no sugars, which means that you are getting 13 grams of complex carbohydrates, which is good. You may consider passing on the item if half or more of the carbohydrates came from sugars. For this to be true for this item, the sugars would have to be 7g or more.

4. Finally, if you are examining a bread product, there should be at least two to three grams of fiber and a couple grams of protien.

If you just ran to your cupboard and found items that you thought were healthy actually contain chemicals, additives and preservatives, you may be thinking that there is nothing you can eat when following these guidelines. Remember they are just guidelines, and yes, sometimes it is impossible to find all food items produced in a healthy way. Rice pilaf is going to be hard to come by with less than 20% Daily Value of sodium. The real lesson here is in food choices. When you go to the grocery store, there will be five to twenty different types of crackers. Choose the best one out of the options. The one you choose does not have to be created perfectly, but make sure it is the best out of your options.

Should I go organic?
After reading the last few chapters about how chemicals, preservatives and artificial ingredients can have an impact on your body and a huge impact on a developing baby, this is a good question. I would first like to explain what *organic* is exactly. Organic foods, as defined and regulated by the U.S. Agriculture Department (USDA), are grown and produced without pesticides, synthetic or sewer fertilizer, antibiotics and are not irradiated or genetically modified. The word organic does not mean healthy; it refers to how something is produced. High fructose corn syrup and pop tarts can be produced organically; you should still avoid eating them. There is no question that organic foods are better for the environment, and that organic tomatoes are healthier and taste better than non-organic tomatoes. Organic food is usually a bit pricier. When you stop buying items off the *Cut the Crap* list, that money

can be put towards organic food. If you can afford to go completely organic, do it. If not, try to buy certain organic items to reduce your exposure to chemicals. The following foods often contain the highest levels of chemicals: milk and cheese, soy products, corn and corn products, apples, applesauce and apple juice, potatoes, peanut butter, spinach and pork. When the time comes, you should only buy organic baby food packaged in glass, not plastic. At the very least, you need to wash all your fruits and vegetables to reduce the amount of chemicals on the outside of the produce.

Give Me A Break

Okay, give the poor pregnant lady a break. Did I leave any room for indulgences during pregnancy? Of course! I have a sweet tooth myself and I can rationalize some treats with a nutritional argument. My number one pregnancy indulgence was ice cream. I was always hot while pregnant, so the cold cools you off. Do not buy sugar free or fat free ice cream. Real sugar is replaced with chemical sweeteners and fat is substituted by adding additional sugar. I feel ice cream is a wise pregnancy indulgence because it is high in calcium and the glycemic load for ice cream is surprisingly low. That is, provided that you don't buy an ice cream that has been loaded up with crushed candy bars or caramel swirls. I recommend getting an all-natural vanilla or chocolate and slicing bananas or strawberries on top, sprinkle with raw nuts and you have made a smart Mommy Fabulous dessert choice.

I also recommend fruit pie as a dessert option. I am not talking about the junk in the metal tin with the clear plastic cover that you find at most supermarket bakeries. Those things are filled with trans fat, high fructose corn syrup, bleached flour and fake berry-colored gel filling. I am talking about an actual fruit pie filled with real fruit. Do they look like actual apple slices? Are there real, whole berries in there with no jelly filling? The best places to find real fruit pies is in organic grocery stores, farmers markets and independent bakeries (not within a larger chain store) or make one yourself. Try to find a bakery that will make you a reduced sugar pie, but not substitute the sugar with chemical sweeteners. When making one yourself, cut the sugar the recipe calls for in half; you will not notice. The flavor of actual fruit is nice when it is not hidden by excess sugar. Not a pastry chef? A nice short cut is to make a topless pie. Just use a pie crust on the bottom and you don't have to worry about baking the perfect crust. See my Mommy Fabulous recipe section for instructions. Fruit is filled with many vitamins and berries, especially, are high in antioxidants.

Frozen fruit bars made of 100% fruit and fruit juice are also a smart dessert option. You need to read the nutrition label carefully because manufacturers put eye catching labels on the front of boxes that can be deceiving. You can also make your own using a popsicle mold. Fill the molds with low fat yogurt and frozen berries or chopped fruit. Try making frozen fruit bars with peach yogurt and chopped peach chunks.

Super Mom - Super Food

I feel that the avocado is the perfect fruit for the pregnant body. Yes, avocado is a fruit. One ounce of avocado contains nearly 20 nutrients your body needs, including vitamins, minerals and phytonutrients, which may help prevent many chronic diseases.[25] Avocados are a great source of monounsaturated fatty acids which are known to be important for the growth and development of a baby's central nervous system and brain. Avocados contain oleic acid, a monounsaturated fat that may help lower cholesterol.[25] This is where you should be getting your dietary fat from…not junk food! Avocados are also high in fiber and enhance the body's ability to absorb fat-soluble vitamins from other foods they are eaten with. Avocado should be used on foods instead of mayonnaise, sour cream or cheddar cheese for flavor and has superior health benefits. Don't buy packaged guacamole or avocado spreads as they are full of preservatives. Avocados are a *real* treat. They cost the same amount, if not less, than a cup of black coffee and do wonders for the body, skin and mind. I would also list raw almonds and berries as being super foods for similar reasons.

Making Healthy Food Choices

This chapter focuses on positive food choices. Let's revisit the *Cut the Crap* list, which told you what items to avoid, but this time let's focus on the added column which gives you healthier substitute suggestions. There are so many wonderful flavors in the world; I know you and your family will find new favorites.

All crap can be substituted with a perfectly acceptable alternative.

Crap	Healthier Substitute
Mayonnaise	Mustard, honey or spicy mustard, avocado
Gravy	Low sodium meat marinades, spice rubs
Whipped cream	Low fat vanilla yogurt
Sour cream	Salsa or hot sauce, avocado
Canned fruit, vegetables or soup	Fresh veggies and fruit, homemade soup
Foods that have been artificial colored	Natural colored foods
Foods that have artificial sweeteners	Natural fruit flavors, sugar, molasses
Foods containing high fructose corn syrup	Sugar, honey, corn syrup, 100% maple syrup
Foods that contain trans fat or hydrogenated oils	Ingredients with no hydrogenated oil
Caffeine	Decaffeinated or caffeine-free
Mocha, frappuccino	Blend black coffee, chocolate soy milk, banana, ice
Coffee creamers	Non-fat milk and sugar
Soda	Mineral water, carbonated 100% juice
Flavored water, sport drinks	Water with lemon, lime or citrus slices
White bread products	Whole wheat, whole grain, oat bran, barley
Sugar cereal	Whole grain cereals
Scones or muffins or bread with frosting on top	Unfrosted, bran or wheat scones or muffins
Pastries	Homemade banana bread, 100% fruit pie
Doughnuts	Whole wheat bagel with low fat cream cheese
Fake fruit gel filling in pies or pastries	Pies made with real fruit
Fried food	Baked, sautéed, grilled foods
Chips	Whole wheat crackers, no salt corn chips
Candy bars	100% fruit leather, granola bars
Processed or cured meat	Fresh fish, poultry or lean cuts of meat
Fast food	Deli or carver sandwich, prepared salads

The Concept of Identifiable Dishes

Identifiable Dishes is a concept I developed while pregnant to help me judge and track my servings. I prepared dishes at home and ordered dishes at restaurants that looked closest to the way food comes naturally. The more processed a food item is from its original form, the more nutrients are lost from that food and the less you know about its ingredients. Chicken, mashed potatoes and gravy is an example of a restaurant dinner with unidentifiable ingredients. Is the gravy from a packet? Is it made from baking grease? Was additional salt added? Were they real potatoes that were mashed, or were they out of a box? Did they mix butter or sour cream into the potatoes? You don't know. The only thing that can be identified is the chicken. An example of an Identifiable Dish would be a Cobb Salad. I can visually identify every food item in the salad and physically separate them into food groups. The more *prepared* a dish is, the less likely you are going to be able to identify exactly what you are eating. An Identifiable Dishes policy involves less time to prepare meals, and you have a perfect excuse not to spend hours slaving in the kitchen…you are pregnant! Adopting an Identifiable Dishes policy will make you better able to accurately judge whether you ate five servings of vegetables today.

Chapter 5

Mommy Fabulous Cookbook

Standing over a hot stove cooking gourmet meals was not one of my priorities while pregnant, even though eating well was. The part I found, and still find, so time consuming is that to make a balanced dinner, you have to cook a main dish and two side dishes. I didn't have that kind of time or energy, and still don't. If I felt like cooking one thing, I would only be eating a chicken breast for dinner, and that is not a well rounded diet for a pregnancy. I perfected some amazing recipes while I was pregnant to solve the dinner dilemma. These recipes are easy to make, gourmet in taste, one dish meals. Some of them are called salads, but believe me, they are not light in calories or flavor. These dishes are substantial enough for you and your spouse to fill up on. I promise none of them will take more than 15 to30 minutes hands on time…but don't tell anyone that! When your husband walks in the door, act tired. Tell him that even though you are pregnant you went to the trouble of cooking this gourmet meal. Hopefully he will tell you how Mommy Fabulous you are!

Dinners

Chicken, Avocado, Mango Rice Salad
Serves 4

1½	cups white jasmine rice
4	boneless, skinless chicken breasts
4	mangos, peeled and cubed
1	large avocado peeled and cubed
¾	cup red onion, chopped
1/3	cup olive oil
1¼	teaspoon salt
¾	teaspoon ground pepper
3½	tablespoons lime juice

Instructions

a. Cook rice until just done according to package directions, omitting salt.
b. Coat the chicken with 1 Tablespoon olive oil, ¼ teaspoon salt and pepper. Cook until done on a grill, or on stove set at medium-high in a grill pan. When chicken is cool enough, cut into ½ inch cubes. (Chicken can be cubed first, then cooked in a wok or frying pan.)
c. Combine rice, chicken and remaining ingredients in a bowl. Serve warm.

Salmon over Orzo Salad
Serves 4

4	salmon fillets (about 1½ pounds)
1	cucumber, peeled and cubed
10	cherry tomatoes, halved
1	cup Orzo pasta
1/3	up olive oil
2½	tablespoons lemon juice
1 to 2	teaspoons dill spice
	black pepper

Instructions

a. Slice cucumber and tomatoes into 1/2 inch cubes.
b. In a pot of boiling water, (do NOT add salt) cook orzo until done, about 12 minutes. Drain. Rinse with cold water and drain again.
c. Toss orzo with 1/3 cup olive oil, dill, lemon juice, ¼ teaspoon salt, 1/8 teaspoon pepper. Add tomatoes and cucumber cubes.
d. Coat salmon with 1 Tablespoon olive oil, 1 Tablespoon dill, 1/4 teaspoon salt and 1/4 teaspoon pepper. Grill salmon until done. Or bake, covered, in oven at 350 degrees for 15 minutes, until done. Splash with 1 teaspoon lemon juice. Serve salmon on top of orzo salad.

Mommy Fabulous Cobb
Serves 4

4	sliced hard boiled eggs, omit 2 yolks
4	tomatoes cut into wedges
2	avocados, cubed
4	grilled chicken breasts
	mixed baby greens salad lettuce
Lemon or balsamic vinaigrette	

Instructions

a. Combine ingredients in a bowl, toss and enjoy!

* You may think there are some ingredients missing here, but pregnant women should not eat soft cheeses and no one needs bacon.

Turmeric Toss
Serves 4

1½	cups white jasmine rice
2	large stalks broccoli, cut into florets (about 7 cups worth)
1	russet potato, cut into ½ inch slices
¾	cup yellow onion, diced
1	15 oz. can diced tomatoes, drained
2	tablespoons olive oil
¾	teaspoon turmeric
1/3	cup water
¾	teaspoon salt

Instructions
a. In a large, deep frying pan, heat 1 Tablespoon oil over medium heat. Cook onions, stirring occasionally, about 5 minutes. Add potato slices and 1 Tablespoon oil. Cook until potatoes are desired doneness.
b. Add broccoli, tomatoes, water, salt, turmeric and bring to a simmer. Reduce the heat and simmer, covered, until broccoli is done, about 10 minutes.
c. Cook rice according to package directions, omitting salt.
d. Serve Turmeric Toss over rice or as a side dish.

Most Fabulous Tacos Ever
Serves 4

1	28 oz. can crushed tomatoes
1	4 oz. can diced green chilies
1	15 oz. can kidney beans, drained
2	15 oz. cans black beans, drained
¼	cup chopped yellow onion
1	package corn tortillas
	olive oil

Instructions
a. Place first five ingredients in a large pot set on moderate heat.
b. Place 1 teaspoon olive oil in a pan. Place corn tortilla in pan and cook on medium-high until tortilla is supple and won't crack when bent in half.
c. Spoon ingredients into tortillas, fold in half, enjoy!

*I was never a fan of corn tortillas. Trust me, try this recipe and it will be one of your favorites.

Baked Maple Chicken
Serves 4

1	package chicken thighs (about 8)
1	yellow onion, cut in ½ inch wedges
2	yams, peeled, cut in 2 inch cubes
2	tablespoons olive oil
1	teaspoon salt
3	tablespoons 100% maple syrup
1	teaspoon thyme
¼	teaspoon black pepper

Instructions
a. Heat oven to 400 degrees.
b. Rinse chicken thighs and cut off all extra fat.
c. Place chicken, onion and yams in a 9 by 13 inch baking dish. Coat with olive oil and season with salt and pepper. Toss. Drizzle maple syrup over top and sprinkle with thyme.
d. Bake covered for 1 hour and 15 minutes.
e. Cool 10 minutes before serving.

*Don't use any syrup; most of them are crap. Use a real 100% maple syrup. It will be more expensive but the taste is amazing!

Bell Pepper Penne
Serves 4

1	16 oz. box Whole Wheat Penne
1	zucchini, sliced, then halve slices
1	red onion, diced
1	red bell pepper, cut into 2 inch strips
1	yellow bell pepper, cut into 2 inch strips
4	boneless, skinless chicken breasts (chicken is optional)
¼	cup White Balsamic Vinegar
1/3	cup Sun Dried Tomato Pesto
¼	cup olive oil
¾	teaspoon garlic salt, or to taste
1	teaspoon dry basil or ½ cup fresh
¼	teaspoon black pepper
½	cup grated Parmesan cheese

Instructions

a. In a pot of boiling water, cook penne, Do NOT add salt! Should take 10 minutes, then drain.
b. Cube chicken breasts. Add 1 Tablespoon olive oil to wok or frying pan. Add chicken, season with ¼ teaspoon salt and 1/8 teaspoon pepper. Cook chicken until done. Or you can grill chicken and vegetables.
c. Add zucchini, bell peppers and 1 Tablespoon olive oil to chicken and cook over moderate heat until tender.
d. In a large bowl, combine penne, vegetables and chicken. Add pesto, olive oil, vinegar, garlic salt and pepper. Toss to coat.
e. Stir in Parmesan cheese, serve hot or chill for an hour.

*If you don't like the taste of whole wheat pasta, this is a good recipe to use it in. You can't taste the difference.

Spanish Spiced Chicken
Serves 4

4	boneless, skinless chicken breasts
2	teaspoons chili powder
1	teaspoon garlic powder
½	teaspoon oregano
½	teaspoon cumin
½	teaspoon salt
¼	teaspoon pepper
¼	cup salsa or picante sauce
	Spanish Rice

Instructions

a. Heat oven to 350 degrees.
b. Place chicken in an oil coated baking dish.
c. In a small bowl, mix chili powder, garlic powder, salt, oregano, cumin and pepper.
d. Sprinkle mix over all sides of chicken and bake covered for 25 minutes or until chicken is cooked through. Spoon ¼ cup salsa or picante sauce over the top of chicken and cook 5 more minutes.
e. Make Spanish Rice. If using a box mix, omit butter and salt additions.
f. Serve chicken on top of rice.

*It is healthier to make Spanish Rice from scratch. If you choose to buy a box mix, choose a brand with the best nutrition label.

California Style Tostadas
Serves 4

4	boneless, skinless chicken breasts
4	naval oranges, peeled, cut into cubes
2	15 oz. cans low sodium black beans
4	soft taco size flour tortillas
1	tomato, diced
1	avocado, sliced into ¼ inch strips
1	tablespoon orange juice
½	cup salsa

Romaine lettuce, shredded

*Option: marinate chicken in ½ cup salsa and 2 Tablespoons orange juice for 1 hour before grilling for added flavor.

Instructions
a. Heat oven to 400 degrees.
b. Season chicken with ¼ teaspoon salt and ¼ teaspoon pepper, then grill. Slice into thin strips.
c. In a bowl, mix salsa with black beans and 1 Tablespoon orange juice.
d. Place tortillas on a cookie sheet and spoon bean mixture on top and add grilled chicken slices. Place sheet on center rack and toast tostadas for 4-5 minutes or until edges begin to lift and tortilla is crunchy. The tortillas should bake stiff like little pizzas, not floppy like a burrito.
e. Top tostadas with lettuce, tomato, orange cubes and avocado slices. Pick up whole tostada and eat like a pizza slice.

Orange Grove - Avocado Salad
Serves 4

4	boneless, skinless chicken breasts
1	any fajita marinade, bottle or spice packet

Romaine lettuce

2	naval oranges, large, peeled, cubed
1	avocado, peeled, cubed
2/3	cup diced red onion

Dressing

1/3	cup olive oil
1/3	cup orange juice
2	tablespoons lime juice
1	tablespoon honey
1	teaspoon garlic powder
½	teaspoon chili powder
¼	teaspoon salt
¼	teaspoon pepper

Instructions
a. Combine chicken, marinade, orange juice and olive oil in a sealed food storage bag and refrigerate overnight.
b. Grill chicken. Slice into thin strips.
c. Mix salad dressing in a small bowl.
d. Combine all ingredients and dressing in a large bowl.
e. Serve.

Dreamy Veggie Sandwich

Serves 2

2	whole wheat sandwich rolls
	Neufchâtel or 1/3 less fat cream cheese
1	avocado, mashed
1	tomato, thin round slices
	fresh spinach leaves
1	cucumber
1	red onion, sliced into thin rings

Instructions

a. Spread cream cheese on top side of roll.
b. Spread mashed avocado over cream cheese.
c. Cut cucumber lengthwise into thin strips, trim to roll length.
d. Generously stack all ingredients in sandwich.

*Don't omit an ingredient because you don't care for it. These veggies really work together here!

Breakfast

Mexican Scramble

Serves 4

6	eggs, pasteurized
¼	cup non-fat milk, pasteurized
1	chili pepper, diced or sliced
1	large avocado, sliced
salsa (choose a thick one)*	
4	slices whole wheat bread
¼	teaspoon salt
1/8	teaspoon black pepper

Instructions

a. In a medium size bowl, whisk eggs, milk, salt and pepper.
b. Add eggs and chili pepper to frying pan and scramble eggs hard.
c. Arrange eggs on a plate and spoon desired amount of salsa over the top. Top with avocado.
d. Serve with whole wheat toast.

*Choose a salsa with corn kernels and tomato chunks so all the flavor is not from added salt or additives. Green bell pepper can be substituted for the chili pepper for less spice.

Mommy's Balanced Pancakes

honey wheat or oat bran pancake mix	
1	sliced banana
½	cup blueberries (fresh or frozen)
¼	cup chopped walnuts
wheat germ	

Instructions

a. Lightly grease and heat griddle on medium heat.
b. Prepare pancake mix according to package instructions.
c. Fold banana slices, blueberries and walnuts into batter.
d. Pour ¼ cup batter per pancake.
e. While cooking first side, lightly dust uncooked top side with wheat germ.
f. Cook pancakes for about 1 and a half minutes on each side or until golden brown.

Dessert

Mother Nature Cookies

½	cup butter
¾	cup sugar
1	egg
½	teaspoon vanilla extract
½	teaspoon baking soda
½	teaspoon salt
1½	cups whole wheat flour
1	teaspoon ground cinnamon
1	cup quick oats
1¼	cup zucchini, grated
1	cup walnuts, chopped
1	cup semisweet chocolate chips

Instructions
a. Heat oven to 350 degrees.
b. In a large bowl beat butter until soft, add sugar and beat until fluffy.
c. Add egg and vanilla, beat well.
d. In a different bowl, whisk flour, cinnamon, baking soda and salt.
e. Set mixer to low, gradually add flour mixture to butter mixture. Beat until blended.
f. Stir in the rest of the ingredients by turning the mixture over itself with a large spoon. Don't over-stir or the oats will break down.
g. Place dough balls 2 inches apart on a cookie sheet. Bake 10-12 minutes.

Topless Apple Pie
1 Pie

1	ready made dough or pie crust
1/3	cup sugar
8	Granny Smith apples, medium
½	teaspoon cinnamon
½	teaspoon nutmeg
	dash salt

*It may be challenging to find a pre-made, all natural pie crust, but they do exist. Look at specialty grocers or online.

Instructions
a. Heat oven to 425 degrees.
b. Place one of the thawed ready made pie crusts into bottom of a 9 inch pie dish.
c. Mix sugar, cinnamon, nutmeg, and salt in large bowl. Stir in apples.
d. Pour apples into pie dish. Roll pie crust edge inward over apples. Place foil around pie dish edge to keep crust from burning.
e. Bake 40 minutes or until crust is golden brown. You may want to take the foil off for the last 10 minutes to brown crust edges.

Mommy's French Pastry
1 Galette

1	ready-made pie crust dough
1/8	cup sugar
3	peaches (fresh or frozen)
½	cup blueberries (fresh or frozen)
1	tablespoon 100% fruit apricot preserves

*Thaw frozen fruit to avoid a soggy crust.

Instructions
a. Heat oven to 400 degrees.
b. Place one thawed pie crust on a baking sheet.
c. Mix sugar, blueberries and peaches in a large bowl.
d. Arrange fruit in a thin layer in the center of the pie crust.
e. Fold pie crust edge inward over fruit. Folded edge will be about ½ - 1 inch wide.
f. Spread preserves over folded crust edge.
g. Bake 15-20 minutes, until crust is golden brown.

Chapter 6

Pregnancy Problem- Food Solution

Is there anything I can do for nausea or morning sickness?

Morning sickness is thought to be caused by an increase of pregnancy hormones, which is completely natural and can be a sign of healthy hormone levels. Sometimes nausea is not caused by pregnancy hormones, but by easy to make, avoidable behaviors. A few mistakes that can make you feel unnecessarily nauseous include allowing yourself to become hungry, taking prenatal vitamins on an empty stomach, getting dehydrated, eating too much sugar and refined grains or becoming overly nervous about parenthood. Always keep a snack in your purse, eat and drink water regularly, eat well according to this book and talk about your fears or concerns about pregnancy and motherhood. Not getting enough sleep can make nausea worse. Finally, many women report that regular exercise improves nausea.

Every pregnant woman who has morning sickness usually tries a couple of things before she finds something that alleviates nausea. In many cases it can't be avoided completely. Try a few of these food remedies:

- Ginger has been clinically proven to relieve nausea. It can be taken in capsule form (do not exceed 1 gram per day) or you can drink it as a tea. You may be able to find ginger candies. I recommend using it as a spice first. Buy ginger root and grate it into your dinner. You should take no more than 3g of grated raw ginger a day. In one clinical trial of pregnant women with severe nausea and vomiting, 250mg of powdered ginger root taken four times a day significantly reduced their discomfort. According to these researchers, ginger is one of the best anti-nauseants available.[26]
- Vitamin B6 has also been shown to reduce nausea clinically. It can be taken as a supplement or can be obtained from foods. Bananas, brown rice, lean meats, poultry, fish, avocados, whole grains, corn, and nuts are all high in vitamin B6.
- Eat crackers before getting out of bed in the morning. Keep a bag of unflavored crackers on your nightstand and eat a few before getting up.
- Eat many small meals rather than larger ones.
- Red Raspberry Leaf tea is very high in an assortment of nutrients including calcium, iron, and B vitamins; all of which are important during pregnancy.
- Peppermint or Spearmint tea, candies or as aromatherapy may improve nausea.

Some nausea remedies may make your particular nausea worse. My advice is to try exercise, eating small portions, and foods high in vitamin B6 first, as these solutions are less likely to aggravate anyone's nausea. Sea sickness wrist bands, found in pharmacies, can also help. If those options don't help, then try ginger, red raspberry leaf tea, peppermint or spearmint. You may hear about other herbs or teas for morning sickness, but I warn you to be careful. Many teas contain caffeine, and herbs and herbal teas can have side effects just like drugs. Some herbs cause side effects like uterine contractions or altering hormone levels in pregnant women. Further, the manufacturing process is not FDA regulated, which means that some herbs can have contaminates in them. While this may not be common, my feeling is that pregnancy is not the time to experiment with herbs.

I am so nauseous and I keep vomiting. I can't keep anything down. What should I do?

The most important thing is to not allow yourself to become dehydrated. Severe dehydration can land you in the hospital with an IV to replace fluids. Sip water or juice often. If you can't keep food down, there is no sense in worrying about a balanced diet. Eat whatever it is that you can keep down, even if it is just bread or rice. It is better to get calories than nothing at all. Your baby will take the nutrients it needs from your body stores and when morning sickness passes, (usually week twelve to fourteen) you will be able to replenish yourself. You may have a condition called hyperemesis gravidarum, a severe case of morning sickness. If you really can't eat anything without vomiting you should call you provider immediately to discuss the situation.

I have constipation! Help!

Another one of the lovely side effects of pregnancy. Pregnancy hormones (progesterone) in the blood stream cause smooth muscles to relax. This happens so that the body can expand for the growing baby. Unfortunately, progesterone is not selective and the smooth muscles of the intestine also relax. This results in decreased intestinal motility which basically means it takes your body longer to push food through and this can cause constipation. You may have different bowel patterns (time of day, number per week) than when you were not pregnant. Medically, constipation means that a person has three bowel movements or fewer in a week.[27]

One cause of constipation can be too little fiber in the diet. To avoid constipation eat dried plums or prunes, figs, dates and raisins on a regular basis. I was so afraid of getting constipation because it can be painful, that I got into the habit of eating one dried plum a day. They are very sweet (nature's candy) and they now come individually wrapped so they can travel with you for a snack. Make sure you are eating whole grains and lots of fruit and veggies. If you are following this book, too little fiber should not be the cause of your constipation. Daily exercise keeps *things* moving as well, so don't skip workouts. People who start a new exercise program often forget they need to increase their daily water consumption, not just during a workout. Dehydration can be a major factor in constipation. Limit foods that have little or no fiber and are high in fat such as cheese, meat, chips, pizza, and processed foods. The following foods are high in fiber:[27]

Fruits: avocado, apples, pears, dried fruit, berries, bananas
Vegetables: spinach, broccoli, carrots, kidney beans
Drinks: fruit or vegetable smoothies
Grains: whole-grain cereal, bran cereal

Finally, don't push when you are on the toilet as this can cause hemorrhoids. Instead practice diaphragmatic breathing described in Chapter 11.

I've heard hemorrhoids are common in pregnancy, how can I avoid getting them?

Hemorrhoids are painful, itchy, enlarged veins in the rectal area. Genetics and age play a role in whether a person develops them. Pregnancy and childbirth put pressure on the area, increasing the likelihood of a rectal vein eruption, but there are many factors that are controllable. Sitting or standing for long periods and gaining too much weight can increase your risk for developing hemorrhoids. Excessive coughing, constipation or hard stools can strain rectal veins. All the advice on avoiding or treating constipation will help to keep stools soft, but diarrhea can be just as aggravating to the anal veins. Heavy lifting can also strain the area. Choose appropriate weights when lifting and don't hold your breath. Exhaling while lifting reduces the body's internal pressure. If you develop hemorrhoids, there are many exercises in this book that will keep you fit without the use of weights. Talk to your doctor about using creams and suppositories to provide relief.

I have gas. I fart occasionally, but it is mostly trapped in my abdomen causing terrible cramps. What can I do?

I know what you are going through; I had two terrible gas episodes. It was so painful! It was just trapped in my body and made my stomach hurt really badly. Slow gastrointestinal motility caused by pregnancy hormones can cause gas. Generally, avoid foods that are high in fat or fried and avoid consuming too much dairy. While different foods cause gas for different people, these are common culprits: [27]

Fats: any fatty or fried foods
Fruits & Vegetables: pears, apples, peaches & beans, broccoli, cabbage, Brussels sprouts, onions,
    artichokes, asparagus
Drinks: soda, fruit drinks, milk, carbonated beverages
Grains: whole wheat, bran
Dairy: milk, cheese, ice cream
Dessert: sugar and sugar substitutes

You can also reduce your chances of getting gas by eating slower and chewing more to cut down on the amount of air you swallow when you eat. Avoid chewing gum, sucking on hard candy, using a straw and jugging when you drink.

I keep getting heartburn, what can I do?

Heartburn doesn't involve the heart; the burning feeling occurs when stomach acid is kicked back into the esophagus, which is located in the middle of your chest. Pregnancy makes you more prone to getting heartburn because the growing baby is pushing on the stomach. As a general rule, large meals and high fat meals stay in the stomach longer, which allows more opportunity to cause heartburn. Spicy foods are also a common cause. Heartburn triggers can vary from person to person, but certain foods and drinks are more likely to cause stomach acid to splash up into your esophagus. These include: [27]

Fats: any fried or fatty foods, corn and potato chips, creamy and oily salad dressings, ground beef,
    fatty cuts of meat, chicken nuggets, potato salad, chicken or buffalo wings
Fruits & Vegetables: citrus fruit, mashed potatoes, raw onion, garlic, tomatoes and dishes
    made with tomatoes like spaghetti marinara and pizza
Drinks: alcohol, caffeine, citrus juices, cranberry juice
Dairy: sour cream, ice cream, regular cottage cheese
Dessert: chocolate, mint flavored foods, high-fat cookies, brownies, doughnuts

If you're prone to heartburn, the National Digestive Diseases Information Clearinghouse recommends that you avoid lying down for three hours after a meal. Sleeping at an incline by raising the head of your bed 6 to 8 inches by securing wood blocks under the bedposts helps reduce heartburn. Elevating your head by using extra pillows will not help.[27]

*Notice that many of these foods also appear on the *Cut the Crap* list. This should not be surprising given my food philosophy. These foods are crap and the body can't function normally on crap. A good illustration of the body not functioning is gas, heartburn and constipation.

I am following this book, and I still have swelling. Is there anything else I can do?

Following the diet recommendations of this book will not guarantee you won't experience any pregnancy discomfort, but it will certainly reduce the number of times you might experience these symptoms or reduce the severity of an episode. If you are following the recommendations of this book, then you are already avoiding high salt foods that contribute to edema. Review these on page 26. While you are pregnant, you don't want to try to reduce swelling by using diuretics (anything that increases the amount of urine produced) such as caffeine, alcohol or medication. There are some natural food solutions that may encourage swelling reduction and won't dehydrate you. The most common foods that work as natural diuretics are watermelon, cucumbers, watercress, artichokes, beets, oats and tomatoes. Exercise can reduce swelling because it increases circulation. Swimming is particularly helpful for swelling. Compression stockings can be helpful if swelling becomes chronic.

I'm drooling, what's up?

Some women experience excessive saliva while pregnant. There is really nothing that can stop it altogether, but eating several small meals rather than larger ones can help. Drink eight, eight ounce glasses of water a day by taking small sips throughout the day. Rinse your mouth with water and spit several times a day so that you aren't always swallowing all the saliva. Chewing sugarless gum can help. Avoid eating a lot of carbs and sour foods which can encourage saliva production.

I am going crazy with cravings for unhealthy foods!

First, make sure you are not obsessing about food all the time. Focus on enjoying the food you are eating rather than day dreaming about unhealthy food. Snack wisely, so you don't get low blood sugar which causes strong cravings. Likewise, avoid foods with a high glycemic index as they can also cause strong cravings. Remind yourself that you do not want unhealthy food and reaffirm your commitment to your health and your baby's. Set a 24 hour rule, or even a five hour rule. If you still crave it the next day, indulge a little, but you will probably be over it. When it comes to satisfying pregnancy cravings, try to choose healthy options that are similar to the unhealthy foods you crave. Refer to the table below to find the item you crave and a healthy substitute. If you can exercise self control, then do so. Buy one truffle rather than a box or a whole bar of chocolate. Sit down and eat it slowly. Enjoy it and move on. Do not buy a box or bag and try to convince yourself that you will only eat one, because inevitably you will eat them all and be left craving more.

Some pregnant women may crave something that is not food, a pregnancy side effect called pica. Do not eat anything that is not food; non-food items often contain substances that are dangerous to you and your baby. Talk to your healthcare provider if you develop pica.

Unhealthy Craving	*Healthy Substitute*
Sugar (candy)	dried fruit, pineapple, yams, sweet potatoes
Salty (chips, pickles)	olives, celery, kale, spinach, chard, seaweed and kelp (as in Japanese sushi rolls, but make sure contents are cooked)
Sour (sour cream, sour candy)	squeeze lemon or lime on dinner, plain yogurt, vinegar dressings or balsamic dip, green apple, pomegranate seeds or juice
Fat (fried food, bacon cheeseburger)	low fat dairy, coconut, olives, avocado, shrimp, fish, comfort foods like stew or casseroles made with lean meat

I feel like I am trying my best to follow your nutrition advice, but I am still gaining a little more weight than I would like. Are there any additional tips you can give me?

First, I would ask you to refer to chapter seven to determine how much weight you should be gaining and when you can expect those gains. If you still feel you are gaining too much, talk to your doctor to make sure there is not a medical situation encouraging weight gain. If everything checks out, here are my recommendations: Under no circumstances should you attempt to lose weight while pregnant. Read chapter three, Clean Burning Fuel, again and do a reality check. Are you really following the advice? Are you really working out as much as you think you are? Are you spending most of your time at the gym zoning out or socializing or actually doing exercises? There are many things not yet discussed that you can do nutritionally to slow down weight gain while still getting all the nutrients you and your baby need.

- Limit mild cheeses. Cheddar, ricotta and mozzarella are so mild in taste that people often use too much, smothering or filling omelets, lasagnas or casseroles with them. Avoid dishes where cheese is the main course such as cheese enchiladas or manicotti. Tell restaurant servers to go light on the cheese, or hold it altogether. You will not be able to tell if your pizza is made with less cheese. Use strong flavored cheeses like Gorgonzola, Parmesan, and Asiago. A little strong flavored cheese will go a long way. Switch from cream cheese to Neufchâtel, which is lower in fat and tastes the same.
- Stop using condiments. Syrup, butter, jam, ketchup, barbeque sauce, and soy sauce add non-nutrient calories and people tend to overeat what they are putting them on.
- Switch from ground beef to ground turkey which is leaner.
- Limit eating out. When you are at a restaurant, order salmon if it is on the menu.
- Stop drinking your calories. Soda, mochas and juice don't fill you up and usually leave you craving more. Plus the extra calories add up. Drink water instead.
- Meal plan in advance for the day or week; plan snacks as well.
- Keep track of your snacks. It is easy to forget how much you have eaten.
- No eating while doing something else. Don't eat while reading, watching TV or working on the computer. People tend to overeat when they are distracted.
- Eat slowly. Meals should take 20 minutes or more. When you eat quickly you are able to overeat before your stomach has a chance to feel full.
- Eat until you are 80% full. Wait 20 minutes before eating fruit if you are still hungry.

These nutritional and behavioral switches will decrease the number of calories you eat either directly or by decreasing tendencies to overeat. Weight should not become an obsession while pregnant. At the same time, there is no reason to gain excessive weight; it puts stress on your body and the baby and increases both your risks for many complications. When you are getting the nutrients you and your baby need, it merely comes down to calories consumed verses calories burned by activity. So exercise!

Do...

Cut the Crap. Make good food choices and you will not have to worry about calories or how much you eat. If you eat a balanced, healthy diet, you will be hungry when you need calories and nutrients and you will feel full when you are full. Drink plenty of water, take your prenatal vitamins, and don't stress.

I have a monster headache, but I don't want to take medication, what can I do?
Headaches are common during pregnancy. There are many non-drug remedies to try:
- Headaches can be caused by dehydration. Start drinking water and it may go away.
- Alleviate tension by taking a long, warm shower or lying down.
- Sleep it off by taking a nap. If you can't sleep, at least close your eyes.
- Meditate by taking long, slow, deep breaths to reduce the pain. This will help you relax, reduce stress and thus relieve the headache. This may be an opportunity to practice pain management skills for labor.
- If you quit drinking caffeine cold turkey, it may cause headaches. Alleviate the pain by taking a small dose of caffeine in a different form than your vice. If you are a major coffee drinker, try

drinking a small cup of caffeinated tea. If you are a big tea drinker, drink half of a soda.

- Try a sensory distraction method by placing your feet in a hot bath and placing a cool rag on your head, or an ice pack on your wrist. I used this pain management technique while I was in labor and it is very effective.
- High or low blood sugar can cause a headache. Make sure you are eating something every few hours to avoid low blood sugar and avoid sugary foods that cause blood sugar to rise quickly.
- Have someone massage your scalp and neck. If no one is around, do it yourself. This worked for me when I had a headache so bad I thought my head was going to explode.
- If headaches are associated with reading you may need brighter light.
- Foods that are known to trigger headaches by constricting blood vessels in your brain are: Alcohol, vinegar, caffeine, chocolate, preserved meats like salami or pepperoni, citrus fruits, yeast, nuts, beans, raisins, soy, and aged cheese. [28]

Avoid headaches by getting plenty of exercise and rest, eating a healthy, balanced diet and avoiding stress. Poor posture can also contribute to getting headaches. Acetaminophen is the safest pain reliever to take during pregnancy. Consult your pharmacist and follow the label instructions. If headaches are severe or you are getting them often, consult your doctor.

I think I am having a migraine, is something wrong?

Some women get migraines for the first time when they're pregnant. These usually occur in the first trimester and are generally caused by hormone fluctuations.[29] Food additives such as nitrates, aspartame and MSG are triggers. Migraines are severe compared to headaches with the pain often localized to one side of the head. Any noise is loud, any light is too bright and you may have visual disturbances. You should call your doctor to discuss treatment.

If you are in your second or third trimester and have a bad headache you should call your healthcare provider right away. It could be a sign of preeclampsia, a serious condition that can become life threatening if not treated. If you've already been told you have high blood pressure, you should call your doctor even if you have a mild headache.

Call your doctor for any unusual symptoms like a sudden explosive headache, a headache that doesn't go away, or if the headache has other symptoms like visual disturbance or vomiting. Call if you have a headache after a fall.

Braxton- Hicks contractions are driving me crazy, what can I do?

Braxton-Hicks (BH) contractions, or false labor, are painless, sporadic, tightening of uterine muscles. These are uncomfortable rather than painful and don't increase in intensity or frequency. They are more common during the third trimester, but some women experience them as early as six weeks while others may never feel them at all. Dehydration can cause muscles to cramp so drinking fluids may cause the contractions to be less frequent or go away. Be sure to visit the ladies room often because a full bladder can trigger contractions. Exercise can help in two ways. Rhythmic breathing, described in this book, decreases BH whereas being sedentary can trigger contractions. If you are experiencing BH and can't exercise, try walking around or repositioning yourself in your chair. Sex can trigger BH in some women because there is a compound in seminal fluid that induces uterine contractions. BH can be annoying, but is nothing to worry about and will go away spontaneously.

I have developed anemia. Is there anything I can do to increase my iron intake?

There are different types of anemia, but anemia developed during pregnancy is usually iron deficiency anemia. This can happen because your body is trying to produce a lot more blood, and you aren't eating enough iron to keep up with demand. You should discuss anemia with your doctor, who may recommend taking additional iron supplements. Supplements, do not always fix the problem, so it is important to do everything you can nutritionally to increase your iron consumption.

There are two types of iron, heme and non-heme. Heme iron is well-absorbed from foods by the body. Foods containing heme iron include beef, poultry and fish. Increasing lean meat consumption is a sure way to get more iron. Eggs, dairy products, fruits, vegetables, grains and nuts provide non-heme iron. The body absorbs both types of iron, but the body's ability to absorb non-heme iron varies depending on other food factors. Here are ways to help your body absorb more non-heme iron:

- Foods high in vitamin C aid in the absorption of iron. Eat citrus fruit and juices, tomatoes, strawberries, melons, dark green leafy vegetables or potatoes with non-heme iron sources to increase overall iron absorption.
- Cooking your vegetables, rather than eating them raw, can increase the amount of available iron.
- Another way to improve the absorption of iron from plants is to include a source of meat which is also iron-rich.
- As demonstrated in a 1986 study from the American Dietetic Association, cooking foods in a cast iron skillet can add significant amounts of iron to your food.
- Eating bran with iron-rich foods decreases iron absorption.
- Calcium can decrease iron absorption. Take your calcium or prenatal multivitamin at a different time than your iron supplement.[30]
- Fiber can decrease iron absorption.[30]
- Tannins (found in tea) and polyphenols (in coffee) can decrease absorption of non-heme iron.[30]
- Eating soy proteins together with non-heme iron sources decreases iron absorption.[30]

I have developed pregnancy induced hypertension; can this be controlled with diet?

It depends how severe your high blood pressure is and how close you are to your due date. Hypertension must be addressed because it can decrease the amount of blood that reaches the placenta, which means the baby gets less nutrients and oxygen. If it is severe, you will need medication. If it is mild you can do a lot to help by eating a very low salt diet. Be sure to drink eight, eight ounce glasses of water per day. Eliminate caffeine, alcohol and processed foods. Exercise daily. When you can, rest with your feet up, or lay down. This lowers blood pressure because the blood does not have to be pumped against gravity.

I have developed gestational diabetes, what can I do?

Gestational diabetes means that you have developed diabetes (high blood sugar) while pregnant. The number one risk factor for developing diabetes is being overweight, which, luckily, you can control. Every pregnant woman should be gaining weight, but excessive or quick weight gain can stress the body.

Gestational diabetes must be addressed by your doctor because many complications can arise such as developing high blood pressure. Your baby is at risk of being born with a high birth weight; making delivery difficult and more dangerous for your newborn. Your baby may have to be treated for low blood sugar after birth or may have problems breathing. While gestational diabetes usually resolves itself after delivery, both you and your baby are at increased risk for Type II Diabetes for the rest of your lives. Every woman is checked for gestational diabetes between weeks 24 and 28 of pregnancy. If you experience extreme thirst, hunger, or frequent urination, mention this to your doctor before week 24.

If you have been diagnosed with gestational diabetes, you should get diabetes nutritional counseling. The American Diabetes Association endorses exercise as a helpful adjunct to a healthy diet.[31] Exercise not only keeps weight in check, but exercise also helps regulate blood sugar levels. You and your baby should continue to follow the advice in this book for the rest of your life to help prolong or prevent developing Type II diabetes later.

I am prone to getting urinary tract infections, how can I avoid them during pregnancy?

A urinary tract infection (UTI) happens when bacteria enter the urinary tract which, unlike the vagina, is sterile and has no natural bacteria. A UTI needs to be addressed by a doctor so that the bacteria don't move up the urinary tract into the kidneys. An untreated UTI can land you in the hospital with a kidney infection which can be life threatening. The best way to keep the urinary tract free of bacteria is to drink eight glasses of water daily so you are flushing the system by urinating regularly. Sugar in the diet can encourage a UTI, whereas an acidic diet inhibits bacterial growth. Eliminate sugars, refined foods and fruit juices as much as possible if you are prone to UTIs or at least when you develop one. Caffeine and alcohol also aggravate the urinary tract. To create an acidic environment in the urinary tract, eat fresh or dried cranberries, drink cranberry juice regularly or take cranberry extract supplements found in pill form in a pharmacy. Any cranberry juice won't do the trick; most contain a small amount of cranberry and a lot of sugar. Look for unsweetened 100% cranberry juice (which is very bitter). Make sure you empty all the urine in your bladder each time you use the bathroom, and never hold it. If you need to go, find a bathroom as soon as possible. UTIs can be treated safely with antibiotics during pregnancy. You must still continue to drink plenty of water, and NEVER stop taking the antibiotics early, even if you feel better.

How can I avoid or treat a yeast infection?

The vagina has a natural balance of bacteria and yeast. A yeast infection occurs when the yeast overgrow. Natural hormonal changes, diabetes, sexual intercourse and antibiotic use can alter the vaginal balance or kill the natural bacteria allowing the yeast to grow uncontrolled. Sugar promotes yeast growth, so limit your intake of sugar and refined foods and juices. You can also eat yogurt containing live cultures of lactobacillus acidophilus, which helps keep yeast growth in check. Keep the genital area clean and dry to decrease your risk of developing a yeast infection. Yeast infections during pregnancy can be treated with creams and suppositories only. Talk to your doctor or pharmacist. If you have a yeast infection at the time of delivery, the yeast can pass into your baby's mouth causing an oral yeast infection called thrush. Don't worry; oral thrush can be treated effectively.

Chapter 7

Weight Gain

Eating for two? I don't think so. You will hear people say this a lot, but a one-month-old embryo is no larger than a sesame seed. You don't need food for two people. In general, a pregnant woman should increase calorie intake by only 300 calories per day, and not until the second trimester.[32] To give you an idea of what 300 calories means in terms of food, an average banana has 150 calories. If you have a cup of whole grain cereal, eight ounces of 2% milk and one banana, you have hit 300 calories. One 16 ounce Berry Lime Sublime smoothie at Jamba Juice has exactly 300 calories. There are 550 calories in a 100 gram chocolate bar. You don't really need to eat that much more food to hit the 300 calorie mark, but you can see how easy it could be to overeat. You may only need an additional 300 calories during the second and third trimester, but you need more nutrients now that you are pregnant. You are probably going to be hungry more often than normal because your metabolism and nutrient needs will be different, especially because you are exercising. Your food choices must be wise so you can pack as many nutrients into those extra 300 calories without having to eat extra food to get all the vitamins and minerals your baby needs. Refer to Chapters 3, 4, 5 and 6 for help on making wise food choices.

According to a study done in 2008, more than one in five women gains excessive weight during pregnancy.[33] In order to ensure you gain the right amount of weight, you first need to determine how much is enough. The first step is deciding if your pre-pregnancy weight was under, normal, or over the ideal weight for your height. Use the chart below to figure out your Body Mass Index or BMI.

Body Mass Index Chart

Find your BMI by locating your height in the left column. Read across the row until you find your approximate weight. Your BMI is the number at the top of that column. A BMI of 20-24.5 is normal. A BMI less than 20 means you are under a healthy weight. A BMI of 25-29.9 means you are overweight. A score of 30 or higher is obese.

Healthy Weight						Overweight					Obese					
Category 19	20	21	22	23	24	25	26	27	28	29	30	31	32	33	34	35
Height (Inches)					Weight (pounds)											
58	91	96	100	105	110	115	119	124	129	134	138	143	148	153	158	162	167
59	94	99	104	109	114	119	124	128	133	138	143	148	153	158	163	168	173
60	97	102	107	112	118	123	128	133	138	143	148	153	158	163	168	174	179
61	100	106	111	116	122	127	132	137	143	148	153	158	164	169	174	180	185
62	104	109	115	120	126	131	136	142	147	153	158	164	169	175	180	186	191
63	107	113	118	124	130	135	141	146	152	158	163	169	175	180	186	191	197
64	110	116	122	128	134	140	145	151	157	163	169	174	180	186	192	197	204
65	114	120	126	132	138	144	150	156	162	168	174	180	186	192	198	204	210
66	118	124	130	136	142	148	155	161	167	173	179	186	192	198	204	210	216
67	121	127	134	140	146	153	159	166	172	178	185	191	198	204	211	217	223
68	125	131	138	144	151	158	164	171	177	184	190	197	203	210	216	223	230
69	128	135	142	149	155	162	169	176	182	189	196	203	209	216	223	230	236
70	132	139	146	153	160	167	174	181	188	195	202	209	216	222	229	236	243
71	136	143	150	157	165	172	179	186	193	200	208	215	222	229	236	243	250
72	140	147	154	162	169	177	184	191	199	206	213	221	228	235	242	250	258
73	144	151	159	166	174	182	189	197	204	212	219	227	235	242	250	257	265

Source: National Heart, Lung and Blood Institute. Adapted from *Clinical Guidelines on the Identification, Evaluation and Treatment of Overweight and Obesity in Adults: The Evidence Report*. U.S. Department of Health and Human Services, 1998.

If you are a healthy weight...

A woman with a healthy weight before pregnancy should gain 25 to 35 pounds during pregnancy. My pre-pregnancy weight was healthy at 147 pounds at a height of 5 foot 8 inches. My goal was to gain 25 pounds. No dieting of course, but a slow controlled gain of 25 pounds was what I was shooting for. I ended up gaining 30 pounds, which was fine and well within the normal range. I delivered right on my due date and about 3-4 of those pounds appeared in the last week of my pregnancy. I include my experience, not for you to compare yourself with me, but because I remember how hard it was to guess what was supposed to happen.

If you are overweight...

Overweight women may need to gain only 15-25 pounds during pregnancy according to the ACOG. Discuss how much weight you should gain during pregnancy early on. Make it clear to your doctor or midwife that you want to gain a healthy amount of weight for your baby's well being, and that you will be eating healthy and NOT dieting to control weight gain. If you're very overweight when you get pregnant, then it's possible you should not add any additional calories to your diet, and it might even be okay if you lose a little bit of weight during pregnancy, particularly if this occurs because you cut out junk food and switch to a healthy diet.[35] If you are completely sedentary and start an exercise program, you may lose a little due to the activity. If you are pregnant and overweight, the important thing to focus on is getting the right nutrients. You will really need to focus on food choices.

If you are underweight...

Underweight women should gain 28-40 pounds during pregnancy. If you are underweight at conception, you may need to add 100 to 300 calories a day during the first trimester just to get you up to a healthy weight and develop vitamin and mineral stores. I do not recommend cutting out activity as a way to retain more calories and therefore gain additional weight. Exercise has many benefits beyond weight control that you don't want to miss out on. Increasing caloric intake is the best way for an underweight woman to get on track. That being said, that does not mean you should add junk food into your diet because it is high in calories. You should choose nutrient dense, calorie dense foods such as whole milk, whole fat dairy, olives, avocados, pasta with meat or veggies and peanut butter.

Gaining weight during your pregnancy is vital to the health of your baby. If you have an eating disorder, now is the time to seek medical attention and treatment. You should not be afraid to gain weight while pregnant, you will lose it after delivery and your baby NEEDS the weight gain to be healthy. If you or your doctor feels that you are an obsessive exerciser, you may not be able to eat enough calories to keep up with your expenditure. You will need to reduce the intensity of your workouts, and limit time spent working out to one hour per day. Use this book as a way to change your workout program so that you can enjoy activity, get appropriate results and gain healthy weight.

If you are carrying multiple babies...

A woman with a healthy weight before pregnancy should gain 35 to 45 pounds if she is carrying twins. Appropriate weight gain should be monitored by your healthcare provider. If you are pregnant with more than two babies, your healthcare provider should make a weight gain recommendation and closely monitor your weight and the development of the babies.

What is the extra weight for?

The average birth weight of a baby born in the US is approximately seven pounds five ounces.[36] So... if the baby weighs only seven pounds five ounces, and you are supposed to gain anywhere from 15- 40 pounds depending on your pre-pregnancy weight, the big questions is where do all the other pounds go?

Approximate breakdown of 30 pounds of weight gain for a person with a healthy pre-pregnancy weight [14]

Pregnancy Associated Anatomy	Weight Gain
Baby	7-8 pounds
Placenta	1-2 pounds
Amniotic Fluid	2 pounds
Uterus	2 pounds
Increase in Breast Tissue	2 pounds
Increase in Maternal Blood	4 pounds
Maternal Water Retention	4 pounds
Maternal Fat and Nutrient Stores	7 pounds

If you are a healthy weight and you gain 30 pounds, the incredible news is that you really only have seven pounds to lose after the baby is born! Some of you may be thinking, *I have spent the last decade trying to lose seven pounds.* You need to remember that if you follow the Mommy Fabulous program, the deck will be stacked in your favor because you will have a better metabolism and better eating habits than you had over the last decade. Follow the program, and I promise you, the seven pounds will melt off and you will have a head start on losing more if that is what you want.

Gaining too little
Now that you know how much your goal weight gain is, I have to stress how important it is to gain this healthy weight. When a woman does not gain weight throughout pregnancy, complications such as premature delivery and/or having a low-birth weight baby can occur.[37] Babies who are born to mothers who do not gain more than 20 pounds are often considered small for gestational age (SGA), meaning they may have been malnourished during pregnancy. They are more likely to develop serious health problems after birth.[38] Do not compromise your baby's health for vane reasons. Trust me, this program works . You can have it all…a healthy pregnancy and a gorgeous body afterward!

Gaining too much
The following are potential problems with gaining too much weight[39]

Gestational diabetes

Varicose veins

Stretch marks

Hemorrhoids

Fatigue

Snorring (can interrupt sleep)

High blood pressure

Shortness of breath during pregnancy

Physical discomfort (backaches, leg pain)

Difficult epidural placement

Increased risk of Cesarean delivery

Cesarean complications (infections, excessive blood loss, operating time greater than two hours)

Risks for the baby include[27]

Stillbirth

Neural tube defects

Difficulty obtaining fetal heart rate

Broken collar bones during birth

Prematurity

High birthweight

Higher rates of childhood obesity

Higher rates of diabetes

The most successful way to avoid these complications is to begin pregnancy at a healthy weight. The next best thing you can do to ensure you gain healthy controlled weight is to pace yourself. Below you will find a guide to help you pace your weight gain over the course of your pregnancy.

Suggested Weight Gain Timeline

If you are a healthy weight...
You should gain no more than three to five pounds during your first trimester. It is perfectly fine if you don't gain any weight during the first trimester. At this time, that tiny baby doesn't need extra calories, but be sure you are eating nutrient dense foods rather than empty calories that processed food provides. During the second and third trimester you should aim to gain about one pound per week.

> When I found out I was pregnant I cut out ALL foods that did not have the highest nutritional content to ensure the healthiest pregnancy and healthiest baby. When I went in for my second appointment, I had lost a pound. That is when I knew I had to get serious about not only eating healthy, but also eating enough. Exercise has its own calorie demands that you are going to need to account for. Not to worry, I just added more calorie-dense healthy foods like all-natural peanut butter.

If you are overweight...
You should aim to gain on the lower end of the 15-25 pound recommendation because you already have enough maternal fat stores. You should gain no more than one to two pounds during your first trimester. If you adopt a healthy diet, cutting out all junk and begin exercising, (which you absolutely should) you may lose a bit of weight during the first trimester which is okay.[35] As long as you are getting your calories from healthy foods and taking prenatal vitamins, your baby should be getting what it needs. You may notice that you can eat more healthy food than junk. Eight ounces of cucumbers has only 14 calories compared with 550 calories in an eight ounce chocolate bar. It's not about dieting; it is about making smarter choices. During the second and third trimester you should increase consumption of healthy calories by 300 per day. You will need to balance that with daily exercise so that you only gain a total of seven to twelve pounds per trimester in the second and third. If you are overweight, your healthcare provider should make a weight gain recommendation and closely monitor your weight.

If you are underweight...
During your first trimester you should gain five to six pounds or more depending on how underweight you are. During the second and third trimester you should aim to gain about one pound per week. If you are underweight, your healthcare provider should make a weight gain recommendation and closely monitor your weight.

If you are carrying multiple babies...
A woman of normal weight before pregnancy should gain 35 to 45 pounds if she is carrying twins. You should gain no more than 3-5 pounds during your first trimester, and it is perfectly fine if you don't gain any. At this time, the twins don't need extra calories, but be sure you are eating nutrient

dense foods rather than empty calories. During the second and third trimester you should aim to gain about one and a half pounds per week.[40] If you are pregnant with more than two babies, your healthcare provider should make a weight gain recommendation and closely monitor your weight.

The best way to gain weight is slowly and consistently.

At one monthly prenatal appointment during my second trimester I found I had gained six pounds. At one pound a week as a guide, I was only supposed to gain four pounds between appointments- yikes! A two pound difference does not sound like much, but when you still have ten weeks to go those extra two pounds would put me over my goal weight gain. So what do you do when you gain too much weight at a certain point in the pregnancy? You NEVER diet! I don't recommend dieting even when you are not pregnant. And you don't stress about it. I simply said to myself, "okay, this month more vegetables, fruit, egg whites and low fat cottage cheese, less peanut butter…. and ice cream." This is not dieting, this is management. You will probably eat more actual food if your choices are less calorie dense. At my next appointment, I had gained two pounds. At one pound a week as a guide, I should have gained four. I never went hungry that month. Over the two month period I gained the exact target weight of eight pounds. I never got on the scale except at the doctor's office. If you weigh in more often, be aware that weight fluctuates from day to day, time of day or what you are wearing. Another reason to avoid the scale between prenatal visits is that you should not start obsessing about weight gain. Once a month is a reasonable length of time to check in on your weight. You don't want to spend all your time thinking about your weight, what you are eating or want to be eating. Just eat smart, exercise often and don't stress about it.

Chapter 8

Exercise is Beneficial During Pregnancy

Here are the incredible, research based reasons I chose to exercise while I was pregnant and feel it is essential for you to exercise too.

Exercise eases morning sickness.[41]

Exercise may seem like the last thing you feel like doing when you don't feel well, but some women report that regular exercise eases morning sickness. Morning sickness can occur at any time of the day. Try exercising in the mornings if you generally get nauseous in the evenings, or vice versa. If you start to feel nauseous, going for a walk might prevent the discomfort from getting worse.

Exercise gives you energy.[41]

This is true for everyone including pregnant women. The number one exercise obstacle during pregnancy is feeling tired. I know I was. However, I know when I worked out I had more energy than when I stayed home with my feet up. I can even say that when I was tired and dragged myself to the gym, promising myself that all I had to do was walk on the treadmill for 20 minutes, I became more energized while I was there and ended up staying longer, returning home feeling better than when I left. So go. On those fatigued days, promise yourself that you only *have* to do something simple, but bring your MP3 player in case you get a second wind.

Exercise will help you sleep better.

The pregnant woman, whether she slept well before becoming pregnant or not, will have less than perfect sleep, at least during the third trimester. When you get in bed, you may not consciously be thinking about how your body is feeling or changing or what clothes still fit or about how your life will change or your baby… but those worries don't just go away. Add in the physical discomfort of sleeping in a new position and you are in for a less than restful night. There is a difference between being physically tired and being sleepy. The pregnant body is often physically tired, but with the mind racing, it often is not sleepy. Exercise will give you energy during the day, but at night you will be ready for bed! You will probably be able to fall asleep faster and sleep more restfully.

Exercise increases skin elasticity.

Elasticity is the skin's ability to stretch. There is much controversy around whether creams and lotions can prevent stretch marks. There is also a genetic factor involved in the likelihood of stretch mark development. What is not controversial is that the skin of a person who works out regularly is more supple and is less likely to damage while stretching. Exercise will help you to gain weight gradually allowing the skin time to stretch. Exercise will also help prevent excessive weight gain, which will, in turn, decrease your likelihood of getting stretch marks. You can't control genetics, but you can exercise, gain weight appropriately and lather up. I used baby oil. You can get stretch marks on the stomach, breasts, hips and butt-anywhere you are increasing in size. I went to bed every night feeling like a glazed ham.

Exercise decreases the risk of developing varicose veins, blood clots and swelling.

Exercise will help you to avoid these common side effects of pregnancy because exercise improves blood circulation. The less you move the more blood pools in your veins. During pregnancy you have a larger blood volume than before. If this large volume of blood is not being circulated through the veins effectively, the valves in the veins can fail under the increased pressure resulting in varicose or spider veins.

Swelling is the accumulation of fluid outside the blood vessels. Excess fluid outside the blood vessels often happens due to poor circulation. Normally, as blood is pumped through an area of the body, this fluid is absorbed into the blood stream and redistributed. If a person stands or sits in the same position for a long time reducing circulation, they may develop swollen ankles or feet. Pregnant women are especially prone to swelling because of the increased fluid volume their body retains. Exercise reduces swelling by improving circulation. Good circulation also decreases the risk of developing blood clots.

Women who exercise while pregnant are less likely to develop complications during gestation, such as diabetes, urinary incontinence and abdominal muscle separation.

Gestational diabetes is diabetes (high blood sugar) that occurs for the first time during pregnancy. Regular exercise improves glycemic control and insulin sensitivity, both of which decrease the risk for developing diabetes. This is true whether you are pregnant or not. In addition, exercise moderates weight gain. Excessive weight gain is associated with increased risk for developing diabetes. For these reasons, pregnant women who exercise are at less risk of developing gestational diabetes. Women who develop gestational diabetes mellitus can often improve their condition through exercise, and such activity is encouraged by the American Diabetes Association.[42]

Diastasis recti is a condition where the abdominal muscles separate. This occurs more often in women who have weak abdominal muscles. Rather than stretching and coping with the increased pressure of the growing uterus, the abdominal muscles pull apart. Core toning and exercise improve abdominal strength.

Due to the pressure the baby puts on the bladder, some women develop urinary incontinence. Women who exercise the pelvic floor muscles are less likely to develop this complication. Pregnant exercisers are also less likely to develop hemorrhoids.

Women who exercise while pregnant experience less discomfort and are more capable of resolving pregnancy related discomfort.

Your body does not normally have another human attached to the front of it. Over the course of your pregnancy, your baby is going to tax your back, shoulders, calves…your whole body is going to try to compensate for the load. Muscles you don't normally use are going to start working overtime. These muscles are going to get fatigued and they are going to get knots in them and it will get uncomfortable. Regular exercise and stretching will keep your muscles loose. Working out loosens up muscles while at the same time toning them. Contrary to what you might think, exercising muscles in addition to the normal work they are doing to help you carry a baby will make them stronger and more capable of doing their job as opposed to more fatigued and less capable.

People who workout are more in-tune with their muscles. A pregnant woman who does not workout is more likely to think, *my back hurts I am going to lie down*. A pregnant woman who is regularly active is more likely to think, *the right side of my lower back is tight, I know the exact stretch that will make it feel better*. This example illustrates how an active pregnant woman is better able to identify the cause of discomfort and understand enough about her body to know how to alleviate it. For the non-active pregnant woman, the discomfort is more likely to last longer and more likely to return because she is not addressing the cause. I am not saying that rest is not a good idea, of course it is, but it is important to recognize that sitting on the couch watching TV and sitting on the floor watching TV while reaching for the ceiling are BOTH resting.

Exercise improves posture.

People who exercise generally have better posture. Poor posture is usually due to poor muscle tone and a lack of trying. The muscles that are supposed to hold a person upright are weak and the person slouches. Weak stomach muscles are a common reason for poor posture and resulting backaches. Posture is especially important for pregnant women because as their abdominal muscles stretch, they overcompensate with their lower back muscles and become more prone to backaches. Posture for a pregnant woman is a nine month transition. Everyday your body is changing, and adapting a new form. It is important to keep postural muscles in shape otherwise you may end up with chronic backaches or headaches near the end of your pregnancy. Exercise prepares the body for extra weight gain. Maintaining or developing good muscle tone enables the body to carry third trimester weight without necessarily feeling weighed down.

Women who exercise are more prepared for the rigorous workout of giving birth.

Women who workout while pregnant are training their bodies in ways they may not even realize. The first way exercise prepares you for birth is through practiced breathing. Focused exercise incorporates controlled breathing in sync with the contraction of muscles. Breathing techniques are the most tried and true method used during labor. Many people instinctively hold their breath through a hard contraction either during labor or during a biceps curl. Holding your breath during a muscle contraction decreases the amount of oxygen available to the muscle, which reduces the number and ability of muscle fibers to contract. Pregnant women who do weightlifting will have practiced this breathing technique more often and for a longer period of time than any child birthing class would have a person practice. After practicing breathing with contraction during workouts for nine months, or longer if you were active before, breathing through contractions will be second nature. Keep in mind, that during labor you don't really have the time or desire to think through these concepts, so the more trained your body is to deal with stress, the more instinctive it will be to react accordingly. There is a difference between breathing to live and deep breathing through a muscle contraction. Normal breathing is an automatic bodily function done without thought. A person does not even need to be conscious to breath. Deep breathing requires focus; remember that it is instinctive to hold one's breath when a contraction becomes difficult. Deep breathing, practiced while doing aerobic activities such as the stair climber, playing sports or cycling will get your lungs in shape for the fast contraction phase of birth (when contractions are close together) where many women breathe quickly or pant and end up exhausted. Swimming and weightlifting will develop your vital capacity, that is, your ability to take in more oxygen. During the course of a pregnancy, a woman must work harder to breathe deeply because the growing baby crowds the diaphragm.

The second way that physical activity trains your body for childbirth is through the development of stamina and endurance. One of the most recommended activities for pregnant women is walking. Yes walk…but don't walk instead of working out. Walk in addition to working out. While walking is a good activity, it is not the best preparation for the rigors of delivery because it does little to build stamina or endurance. In fact, I could argue that compared to other activities such as swimming or weightlifting, that walking is harder on joints, especially the knees. I also found that during my last trimester, the repetitive low level bounce in the steps of a long walk made my already stretched abs ache uncomfortably (this is a common, temporary effect called lordosis). The same amount of time spent lifting weights, swimming, cycling or stair climbing gave me a better cardiovascular workout and I did not have lordosis (achy lower abdomen) afterwards.

Now if you are thinking that you will just get an epidural and won't have to worry about breathing or having stamina, rethink your position. There are many scenarios where your blissful drugged up birth won't happen. You may get to the hospital too late (road construction detour) and medical staff will determine that you can't get an epidural this late in the game. Some people do not respond to an epidural, or the pain relief is not complete. Sometimes the epidural wears off before the baby is delivered. Some women can not have an epidural due to prior surgeries or spinal deformities they may not even be aware of. There may not be an anesthesiologist available for a while. In each of these scenarios you will still need to cope with pain. Sometimes, women who planned to *not* have to deal with pain become panicked when the drugs don't work. Their perception of pain may be much worse. My advice is to be prepared to give birth naturally. Read some books on pain management and practice the techniques. Get pain relief if you want it during labor, but do not go into the pregnancy and labor expecting to not have to cope with the rigors of childbirth.

Many studies have shown that women who exercise feel labor is easier.[43] Exercise may lower the perception of pain during labor. This may be because exercisers are used to the burn of hard muscle contraction, or the feeling of control over contraction, or the confidence developed by knowing you can power through another two reps. It could be a general build in pain tolerance. When I was in labor, I knew I could handle a two minute contraction. I would ask my husband how much time was left. 30 seconds, I knew I could do it. Labor was definitely UNCOMFORTABLE. But I guess, for me, the difference was that I knew I was capable. I wasn't thinking, o*h God, here comes another one*. It was more like, *okay, here we go, two minutes*.

Studies have shown labor to be shorter in women who exercised than those who did not.[44]

After giving birth, I can honestly say I would rather slave over a stair climber at the gym for thirty minutes while pregnant than spend one extra minute in a delivery room…and my labor was easy compared to other people's labor stories. The incentive of a shorter labor inspired me to get to the gym on many days! Once you are in labor, you will agree that time spent exercising was time well spent.

Pregnant exercisers experience fewer obstetric interventions.

Women who workout while pregnant have fewer episiotomies, artificial rupture of the membranes, epidurals and other pain medication, induced labor, electric fetal monitoring, vacuum extraction or forceps delivery and caesarean section.[45] Exercise decreases the risk of having a normal birth turned into a major medical procedure. Exercise can also protect your baby from delivery complications. Having a heavy baby, associated with excess pregnancy weight gain, increases your risk of having vaginal tears, and the baby can suffer stuck shoulders and broken collar bones.[7]

Women who exercise while pregnant will have an easier time losing pregnancy weight and get back into shape faster than women who didn't exercise while pregnant.

Have you ever heard the saying that it takes a long time to get into shape, but it only takes two weeks to get out of shape? The effects of aerobic training are rapidly lost when activity ceases. Losing weight is infinitely easier if you are already in shape (regarding cardiovascular fitness and muscle tone). If you workout while pregnant, you will be in shape under those extra baby pounds and it will be easy to shed them. Muscle tone and strength are maintained much longer than cardiovascular conditioning, which is why resistance training is the smartest pregnancy exercise choice. Do you think it is it easier for a person to lose weight if they worked out three to seven days a week for the last nine months, or will it be easier for a person who hasn't been to the gym in nine months? This is just common sense. If you think that you will just *deal with* getting back into shape after the baby is born, (i.e. relax now, pay later) I am telling you that is a bad idea. If you think you are tired now, you will be more tired postpartum. If you think you are too busy now, you will be more busy postpartum. If you think chasing a toddler around will help you lose the weight, let me tell you, you won't be able to keep up with a toddler, AND you will be absolutely sick of maternity clothes. Believe me, you will want to burn them as soon as possible and get back into the cute fashions you haven't been able to wear. AND… if I can add just one more reason why you will enjoy a faster, easier, postpartum recovery…you will get all this, "oh my gosh, I can't believe you gave birth only two months ago, you look Mommy Fabulous!" Okay…so they probably won't use the phrase Mommy Fabulous, but I guarantee they will say the first part.

Exercise has psychological benefits for everyone.

Exercise is proven to elevate mood, decrease the risk of developing depression and ease stress and anxiety by releasing feel-good hormones. Exercise improves self esteem because of the sense of accomplishment, not just because you look good. It helps a pregnant woman maintain healthy weight gain which is also something to feel good about. Studies have shown that women who worked out while pregnant reported feeling better about their changing bodies and had a more positive self image.[46] In addition, women who exercised while pregnant had a lower incidence of depression both while pregnant and postpartum.[47] Happy women make happy wives and mothers. Everyone wins when mom works out!

Exercise and Your Baby

Exercise may improve physical development during pregnancy.

The placenta supplies the baby with oxygen and nutrients. Studies have shown that moderate exercise during early pregnancy improves growth of the placenta.[48]

Babies born to mothers who exercise while pregnant may be smarter.

Babies born to mothers who worked out while pregnant were more cognizant and developed faster according to a study that followed newborns through age five. These children scored significantly higher than children of non-exercisers in tests of intelligence and language over the five year study period.[49]

Exercise during pregnancy may improve the future health of your baby.

Exercise contributes to healthy, controlled, maternal weight gain. Uncontrolled or excessive weight gain is associated with having a baby that weighs over nine pounds at birth. Newborns weighing nine pounds or more have a greater risk of developing diabetes later in life and are prone to being overweight.[33] A study that followed newborns through age five found that children born to mothers who worked out while pregnant were leaner through the age a five than the children of women who did not exercise while pregnant. These leaner children had growth within the normal range for their age, but they had healthier body fat.[49]

Are you convinced that exercise is important to your pregnancy? I hope so, but if you still have reservations based on something you heard, read this list of pregnancy exercise myths. Each myth is followed by the truth. There is a lot of misconception and bad advice out there. The following myths are misguided advice you may receive while you are pregnant. Be prepared to set the record straight!

Myths Based on Faulty Scientific Support

MYTH: Blood will be diverted from the placenta to the muscles during a workout putting the baby at risk for hypoxia (oxygen shortage).
TRUTH: A pregnant woman has an increase in blood volume, increased vein capacity and increased hematocrit (oxygen carrying blood cells). These factors mean there is more oxygen available, which would offset a theoretical decrease in oxygen to the baby while exercising.[50]

MYTH: A woman can become too warm while working out and this could cause the baby to overheat.
TRUTH: Women do produce more heat while pregnant. A person also produces more heat while exercising, so the combination of the two sounds like a solid, theoretical risk. However, a woman's body undergoes some adaptive changes during pregnancy. To compensate for the increased heat production, the pregnant body has greater vasodilation at the skin, resulting in greater heat loss and a reduced tendency to overheat (hyperthermia).[51] Wearing loose, breathable clothing and exercising in a well ventilated area will also help. Drink a glass of water before exercising and continuously during

exercise to stay well hydrated. Keep in mind that sweating is a way for the body to cool off; it is not a sign of overheating. As long as you avoid exercising in a hot, humid climate, exercise shouldn't cause your core temperature to rise. However, because birth defects can be caused by raising the maternal core temperature, you need to avoid hot tubs, saunas and steam rooms and seek medical attention for fevers.[52]

MYTH: If you are going to exercise, it should be for a short time and your heart rate should not exceed 140 beats per minute.

TRUTH: This myth is based on old, outdated pregnancy guidelines. Current guidelines from ACOG do not give a time restriction for a workout. Guidelines do recommend that a woman's perceived exertion is mild to moderate. Chapter Nine will explain how to measure perceived exertion. A mild to moderate workout can last as long as the woman feels comfortable. I heard this 140 beats a minute thing when I was pregnant. A friend kept telling me to go out and buy a heart rate monitor. As it turns out, this was the recommendation made in 1985, and this recommendation was made as a blanket statement not based on any relevant studies. There was no prenatal research to base guidelines on at the time, so they were very conservative. To put this into perspective, the World Wide Web was not invented until 1992. 140 beats a minute is super old advice! The most recent guidelines have thrown this recommendation out and have adopted the more appropriate advice that a woman should workout "mild to moderately most if not all days of the week."[14] Forget the heart rate monitor, unless you are concerned that you will not work out hard enough in an effort to keep it moderate.

MYTH: Strength training should be avoided while pregnant.

TRUTH: Strength training is low impact and mildly elevates your heart rate making it a great pregnancy activity. Toned muscles improve posture and are more capable of dealing with physical pregnancy changes. Strength training involves controlled breathing in sync with the contraction of muscles which can prepare you for labor. In fact, strength training is suggested as an appropriate activity for pregnancy by the American College of Obstetrics and Gynecology.[53]

There is a breathing technique called the Valsalva maneuver. It was invented to test cardiac function, but many people do it accidentally while weightlifting. The Valsalva maneuver involves holding your breath or pushing air out against pursed lips. The Valsalva maneuver increases blood pressure temporarily and because a pregnant body already has an elevated blood pressure, this is not a good idea. This type of breathing is the wrong way to breath during weightlifting whether you are pregnant or not. This book will train you to breathe properly, so this becomes a moot point. You should never hold your breath when doing any type of exercise except swimming. Holding you breath underwater is not an issue as it does not raise your blood pressure.

MYTH: Running is contraindicated during pregnancy.

TRUTH: Running programs should not be started, but for the person who enjoys running, continue to enjoy it until it is no longer comfortable. Many professional marathon runners train until they are due, delivering healthy babies. As your baby grows however, the uterus will push into your diaphragm preventing you from breathing deeply. For some women, this causes their performance to decrease and they feel like running is becoming harder. Some women experience no change is respiratory ability. Listen to your body and you will know when it is time to look elsewhere for aerobic exercise.

MYTH: A woman who exercises while pregnant will become exhausted.

TRUTH: As long as you are not exercising at extremely intense levels, you should be fine. With adequate sleep and nutrition, exercise should make you feel more energized. If you feel exhausted, take a day or two to stretch as your workout. If the feeling persists and you feel you get enough sleep and nutrients, then you should consult your physician, as there may be other medical issues present.

MYTH: Laying on your back blocks an artery resulting in less blood flow to the fetus, so you should not do sit-ups while pregnant.

TRUTH: The first part of the myth is true, the second is not. There are blood vessels that run down your back, and if you lie on your back (the supine position) after the forth month, it decreases blood flow. (In medical terms: The aorta and inferior vena cava may be occluded while in the supine position by the increased weight and size of the uterus after the fourth month.) This is the reasoning for advising against exercise in this position. Decreased blood flow associated with the supine position may cause the following symptoms:

- Increase in maternal heart rate
- Faintness
- Nausea and vomiting
- Headache
- Weakness
- Shortness of breath
- Dizziness
- Sweating or cold, clammy skin
- Numbness in extremities
- Restlessness

These symptoms do not develop suddenly from spending a short time on your back. Symptoms are more likely to happen when lying on your back for a longer length of time such as sleeping or watching TV. Spontaneous recovery usually occurs with even a small change in your position. If you feel any of these symptoms while lying on your back, do not suddenly stand up. Changes in position from lying to upright should be done cautiously to decrease symptoms of lightheadedness. Frequent position changes, putting a pillow under your right hip while lying on your back, or elevating the head with several pillows are all ways to decrease your risk for vessel occlusion while lying on your back. As far as ab crunches go, you have four months to strengthen your abs while on your back without risk. I have devised pregnancy modifications for the exercises in this book and there are MANY ways to work your abdominal muscles without lying on your back.

MYTH: Strong maternal abdominal muscles will not give the baby enough room to grow.
TRUTH: Strong maternal muscles will help to promote good posture and help prevent backaches. Competition bodybuilders with ripped abs and defined six packs deliver healthy babies that were in no way inhibited from growing by their mother's ab muscles. Strong ab muscles will keep your waistline smaller, longer into your pregnancy, which may decrease stretch mark development or discomfort. The baby and placenta have plenty of room to grow within the abdominal cavity before having to push outward for space. Women with weak abdominal muscles are more likely to develop diastasis recti, a condition where the ab muscles separate due to the internal force of the growing uterus.

MYTH: The rigors of exercise could cause a miscarriage or preterm labor.
TRUTH: Miscarriage due to exercise really has no scientific basis. The theoretical, scientific concern is that increased hormone (norepinephrine and prostaglandin) output during exercise could stimulate uterine activity and premature labor.[54] Multiple studies have shown no association with preterm birth and exercise in low-risk pregnancies.[55]

MYTH: Exercise may cause a baby to have low birth weight.
TRUTH: There is no conclusive evidence showing exercise to have any effect on birth weight. What seems to be the biggest factor for birth weight is caloric intake. If you eat enough and workout your baby's weight will not be affected adversely.[56] Conversely, if you eat too much and don't workout enough your baby may be large, putting your baby's future health at risk and you at risk for caesarian delivery.

MYTH: You should not exercise because you could get hurt.
TRUTH: Anyone can get hurt doing anything. The most common sited reason for this caution is the theoretical risk that maternal hormonal changes cause increased joint laxity which could possibly result in an increase in the risk of sprains or strains. However, there are no reports showing an increase in

actual injury rates with exercising pregnant women.[57] So at best, this is theoretical. I do encourage pregnant women to be careful while working out, and when crossing the street for that matter. Strong muscles support joints. Women who do stability exercises, such as those described in this book, while pregnant, are less likely to fall or experience lax joints during their pregnancies than women who do not exercise.

MYTH: If you didn't exercise before, you should not start while you are pregnant.
TRUTH: This is the biggest load of crap! Now is the perfect time to make life changes. Stop cursing like a sailor, stop smoking, start eating healthy and start working out! Pregnancy is not an excuse to remain sedentary or gain excessive weight according to the American College of Obstetrics and Gynecology.[56] You're going to be a mother, the most important role model on earth. The time to get Mommy Fabulous is now!

MYTH: You can worry about getting in shape later.
TRUTH: Having a baby changes your whole life. Changes made now are more likely to stick for life than after you have settled into your new family routine. Good luck making life changes after you have gotten your baby hooked on crap food and a lazy lifestyle. Studies are showing that one in five women gain too much weight during pregnancy and the vast majority doesn't lose this weight before they conceive their second baby. After they have finished having children, they have accumulated many extra pounds and the trend is contributing to obesity in the US. Even those who do lose the pregnancy weight are still at a disadvantage. I have tons of clients come to me saying, "I lost all the pregnancy weight, but my stomach has never looked the same." Postpartum recovery to a Mommy Fabulous body is infinitely easier and faster if you do specific types of exercise during pregnancy.

There are still unanswered questions with regards to exercise and pregnancy. All the current research cannot guarantee the absolute safety of every pregnant woman. However, I do feel there are more risks in a sedentary pregnancy than an active one. Listen to your body and make informed decisions. Remember that even though there are a lot of doctor's office visits and tests performed, you are not sick. You are healthy, and pregnancy is a sign of good health. There is nothing wrong with a healthy person staying fit.

Share the information in this chapter with your husband; you will want his support and motivation in the months to come. Then, make sure he reads or listens closely to the following box.

Attention Husbands

Your wife needs you. There is a lot to look forward to now that your wife is pregnant, a new baby, big breasts. But there are some other physical changes that may not be so cool, big belly, big hips. Your wife's physical fitness will make this pregnancy easier on everyone. Less aches for her means less complaining for you to hear about. Make her fitness your priority. Make dinner or do the dishes so she can go to the gym. Be her motivator, be her support system. She will be tired, so you should encourage her to get her walk in for the day. Go with her. Believe me; your commitment to her fitness has its rewards for you. This fitness program is designed to help her bounce back after she has the baby. You will love your hot, fabulous wife's body after she recovers from childbirth. If she does not workout while pregnant, it may be a long hard road to get back in shape afterward, and it will be more difficult to find the time with a baby around.

Chapter 9

Exercise Precautions

You know exercise is important for a healthy life and pregnancy. There are, however, some cases in which women should not exercise. If you have any of the conditions listed below, you should NOT exercise during your pregnancy according to the ACOG.[58]

Risk factors for preterm labor

- Vaginal bleeding after the first trimester
- Pregnancy related hypertension
- Premature rupture of membranes
- Incompetent cervix
- Placenta previa
- Intrauterine growth retardation
- Women carrying multiple babies who are at risk for preterm labor

Women who have **pre-existing medical conditions** (non-pregnancy related), such as heart disease or constructive lung disease should be carefully evaluated by their physician to determine if exercise is appropriate for their circumstance. For a woman with a chronic condition, aerobic or strength training can add additional strain on a pregnancy. At the same time, no activity at all is also ill advised. Women with these conditions should participate in stretching and toning activities such as leg lifts and arm circles performed without weights. These activities can be done while lying down or sitting. These no-impact activities will help a sedentary pregnancy by keeping the body limber in order to prevent or alleviate muscle aches and to improve mood and prevent depression without significantly elevating heart rate. These types of exercises can be found in the Mommy Fabulous Floor Workout on page 101. Discuss options with your doctor. Medical supervision and caution are extremely important for women with serious conditions such as uncontrolled Type 1 diabetes, seizure disorder, or anemia.[14] If you have any chronic disease, you should ask your doctor: "Is there any reason that I should not exercise during this pregnancy?" and "How will my condition interfere with a healthy exercise program and a healthy pregnancy?"

Underweight women should probably be cautioned about vigorous exercise by their physicians because these women bear more premature and low birth weight infants than normal-weight women. Being underweight doesn't necessarily mean you shouldn't exercise while pregnant. You will need to increase your caloric intake and gain extra weight during the first trimester in order to get up to a normal healthy weight.

Overweight women and their babies are at increased risk for many pregnancy complications including gestational diabetes, high blood pressure, and cesarean delivery. Dr. Artal is the chairman of the Department of Obstetrics, Gynecology and Women's Health at Saint Louis University and has conducted numerous studies on obesity during pregnancy. He is an expert in treating high risk pregnancies. Dr. Artal recommends, "…in uncomplicated pregnancies, all women, even those who are obese, should engage in physical activity." He also says that, "There is still a prevailing reluctance among healthcare providers to prescribe lifestyle modification in pregnancy that includes judicious diet and exercise."[35] His research has shown that "Obese pregnant women who engage in physical activities during their pregnancies reduce their risk of developing gestational diabetes by fifty percent."[35] Take this opportunity, while you are motivated, to follow the nutritional advice in this book and make physical activity a priority in your life. If you are overweight, I encourage you to look into the research of Dr. Raul Artal.

Morbidly obese or excessively underweight women should exercise under supervision and with caution. The exercise program described in this book is not designed for an extremely obese person. Many of the individual exercises however, may be appropriate and beneficial.

Women **carrying more than one baby** should get an exercise program that is individualized and medically supervised. This is because women carrying more than one baby are at significant risk for premature labor.[14] The exercise program described in this book is not designed for a multiple gestation pregnancy. Many of the individual exercises however, may be appropriate and beneficial. Check with a healthcare provider before beginning.

If you have no obstetric or medical complications, you should receive the green light to exercise. For those who already exercise, you can continue at close to pre-pregnancy intensity levels.[14] That being said, there are a few activities that are considered off-limits during pregnancy. It's time for some ground rules. All sources agree that these activities should be avoided by pregnant women no matter what their fitness level is.

Activities to Avoid

- Downhill snow skiing is not safe. Your changing center of gravity can cause balance problems. This puts you at risk for severe falls and injuries. Even if you are skilled and careful, some hazards are beyond your control. For instance, exercising at altitudes higher than 6,000 feet can increase your risk of altitude sickness. This makes it harder for you to breathe and may cut down on your baby's supply of oxygen.
- Horseback riding, gymnastics, water skiing, or other activities where there is an increased risk of falling should also be avoided.
- Contact sports such as basketball, ice hockey or soccer are off limits for now. The high likelihood of being hit could result in harm to both you and your baby. Any other activities where you could be hit by someone or something are also not a good idea. Baseball is an example.
- Scuba diving should be avoided during pregnancy. The large amount of pressure from the water puts your baby at risk for decompression sickness.

Signs that Something is Wrong

These are a few physical signs you do not want to ignore. If you develop any of these symptoms stop exercising and call your doctor.

- Muscle weakness. This is different from having sore muscles or fatigued muscles. Muscle weakness is more like muscle failure. For example, you feel weak pouring milk out of the gallon container.

- Calf pain or swelling. Again, this is not a muscle ache, it is actual pain. These symptoms could indicate a blood clot which needs medical attention immediately.
- Chest pain or trouble breathing. If you are still breathing rapidly or can't seem to catch your breath after you have cooled down from a workout, call your doctor.
- Vaginal bleeding. After the first trimester you should not experience any vaginal bleeding. Call your doctor about vaginal bleeding whether it occurs in relation to exercise or not.
- Headache, dizziness or lightheadedness. Headaches can occur for a number of reasons including dehydration. Drink water, sit down and call your doctor if the headache does not go away. If you are lightheaded or feeling faint you should lay down immediately. Low blood pressure often causes lightheadedness. Lying down allows blood and oxygen to reach your brain under less pressure than when your head is above your heart (standing or sitting). Lying down will decrease the chance that you will pass out. It is better to lie down and let your body adjust, than to fall and injure yourself or the baby on the way down.
- Uterine contractions. These could be Braxton–Hicks contractions. Braxton–Hicks are painless tightening of the uterine muscles that do not increase in intensity or frequency. Braxton –Hicks spontaneously disappear and are not cause for worry. If contractions are painful as opposed to uncomfortable and you are close to your due date, you may be in labor. If you are more than three weeks from your due date and contractions continue or get closer together, call your doctor immediately.
- Decreased fetal movement. Sometime during the second trimester you will begin to feel your baby move. You will probably be able to notice a pattern in the baby's active times of day. When I worked out, Talia never moved…maybe she enjoyed the soft bouncing or the music. Afterwards, I could feel her squirming around like crazy. Some babies become very active when the mom is active. My friend Jayme used to joke that Noah was doing kickboxing too, because he moved a lot during class. You should call your doctor whenever you notice a prolonged change in your baby's behavior whether it is related to exercise or not.
- Fluid leaking from the vagina. This is not caused by exercise, but may be noticed only when exercising. There may be a tear in the placenta that is leaking amniotic fluid. If you only notice leaking fluid while working out, it could be that when you are not active the pressure of the baby resting against the placenta could block or plug the tear. When the mother is active, the movement could allow the tear to leak. This needs to be checked by a physician as excess fluid loss is dangerous for the baby. Be aware, that some women experience urine loss while exercising. The weight of the baby along with active bouncing may put enough pressure on your bladder that it causes you to lose a bit of urine. Transient loss of bladder control is not something that indicates that you need to stop working out, nor is it an emergency. It actually suggests that you should do more pelvic floor exercises to strengthen the area.

Make Exercise Safer

Here are a few safety considerations for every exercising person. Always stay well hydrated. Wear a sports bra that provides lots of support to protect your stretching breast skin. Do not wear underwire bras while pregnant, especially not when working out. Wear clothes that breathe. I was always hot while pregnant so I had to be in a tank top and shorts to workout. Do not feel like you have to hide your changing body; wear what is comfortable. Wear shoes that provide enough support. In general, tennis shoes should be replaced every 300 to 400 miles. If you run three miles a day, five days a week, you would need new shoes every five months. You can always compare your tennis shoes to a new pair to see if the soles and support are breaking down. Finally, avoid intense workouts in high altitude or in hot humid weather and don't exercise to exhaustion.

Perceived Exertion

According to the American College of Obstetrics and Gynecology, "If you are active now, pregnancy need not cause you to alter your fitness routine."[14] However, while pregnant, you should not be attempting to set any records. It can be a bit confusing to know how hard is too hard to workout while pregnant; after all, you want to do what is best for you and your baby. During pregnancy, a woman has an elevated heart rate compared to when she is not pregnant. So if you normally measure your heart rate to gauge intensity, you would have to adjust any calculations you have done based on your new resting heart rate. Poor manual heart rate measurement technique can lead to errors, so an electronic heart rate monitor can be more accurate. I don't feel heart rate monitors or manual measures of heart rate are necessary for the average low risk pregnancy. The current ACOG guidelines do not have a recommended heart rate for pregnant exercisers, so I don't feel that a heart rate measurement tells you much. Assessing *perceived exertion* is the best way to monitor your exercise intensity. Perception of effort can be judged on a ten point scale. A one on the scale would be very easy, four to five would be moderate and a ten would be very, rigorously hard. That is, a ten, would be the maximal effort you are capable of, while a one would be the minimum about of activity you could do and still consider it active. Different activities and different intensities will be perceived at different exertion levels by each person. For example, a very fit person who is skilled at kickboxing may put a very vigorous kickboxing workout as a ten. That same person could take the intensity down and kickbox at a five, which would be moderate. An unfit person or someone who has never done kickboxing may put kickboxing at any intensity as a ten. ACOG guidelines recommend that a woman's perceived exertion is mild to moderate. Again, what is mild to moderate for one person may be difficult for another.

Another way to gauge mild to moderate exertion is by doing a **talk test**. You should be able to breathe throughout the entire activity. You should be able to speak a short sentence like, "I need to get a drink," without having to gasp for air. If you can remain conversational during your workout, you are probably at a mild exertion level. Many pregnant women workout at a mild exertion level of one to three when an exertion of four to five is reasonable and safe.

If you feel like you can not accurately gauge your exertion by using the concept of perceived exertion, then a heart rate monitor is a great option. Decide on a heart rate that is a moderate intensity and use the heart rate monitor to make sure you exercise at that heart rate. This strategy can keep you honest. The heart rate monitor will tell you to get the lead out when you are feeling lazy. Without it, you may be able to convince yourself that you are trying when you are really loafing.

Beware of exercise psychology! Some people don't enjoy working out, and with that mentality, an activity can seem hard. A person who hates the treadmill could get on it and feel like two miles an hour is hard (a seven on the perceived exertion scale). If this sounds like you, a heart rate monitor might help. If you feel so tired and that the treadmill is so hard, but see that your heart rate is only 100 beats per minute, you will realize that you may need to increase the speed to four miles an hour to get a moderate heart rate and workout going. Keep in mind that a particular activity may *seem* hard, but the same effort at a different activity may be mild. If the treadmill seems like a drag, take up stair stepping or swimming.

Make sure you consult your doctor before you start any fitness program. I am sure your doctor will give you many cautions, but make sure to ask, "Doctor, is there any reason that I shouldn't exercise during this pregnancy?"

Chapter 10

The Mommy Fabulous Workout Program

Many of my pregnant friends and clients have asked me, "How did you develop the Mommy Fabulous Workout Program?" I developed the Mommy Fabulous maternal exercises based on a lifetime of sports and physiology. With a background in physical rehabilitation and a degree that focused on health and sports medicine, I created a fitness program for my pregnancy that would address all the challenges a pregnant body faces. The philosophy is to minimize the side effects of pregnancy while harnessing the increased metabolic rate that every woman develops while pregnant and reset the body physiology to maintain that metabolism after delivery. This will kick-start your postpartum recovery while you are pregnant. The best way to do this is by maintaining or increasing your muscle to fat ratio while gaining healthy weight, not just packing on body fat during pregnancy.

Why should I switch from my current fitness routine?

The biggest problem with most people's workout routine is that they do what they are best at. People like to do the things they are good at; it makes you feel good about yourself. People with good flexibility do yoga and people with good stamina run. Welcome homeostasis! Doing the same exercise routine is only gong to keep you in the same shape. If you run three miles everyday for ten years, you will probably stay the same weight. Your muscles will get used to the activity, adjust and won't really react until you change something. Always doing the same activities will result in muscle imbalances. Muscles you use often will be stronger than muscles you ignore. This can lead to what is called overuse injuries for the repetitive activities you do. As your body changes during pregnancy, this can lead to aches and pains because ignored muscles are now being strained while stronger muscles are knotting up to overcompensate. A good example is the person who only runs, jogs or walks. As the breasts get heavier, their ignored and weak upper back muscles can't cope and end up aching.

Most people workout incorrectly for their goals. You have a new goal: minimizing the negative effects of pregnancy and looking hot after delivery. I doubt your old routine or sport is designed to deliver this result. Poor exercise choices, poor form, monotony, lifting too fast or using too much weight can lead to injury and no real results. If you exercise smart, it will take you less effort to stay fit. I am going to show you how to do this. I am going to coach you on form and mix up your workout. I am going to challenge your weaknesses, not ignore them. This program is designed to keep you safe while your body is changing. You will not get ripped, or get into amazing cardiovascular shape- come on, your pregnant. You will gain weight and your waistline will only increase. The secret here is that you can remodel your body while you are pregnant by taking advantage of the changes that are going on so that you will recover from your pregnancy with a kick ass Mommy Fabulous body faster than you thought possible. There is a small window of time (nine months) to take advantage of this opportunity. You will be able to wear a bikini by summer if you deliver in February! If you follow this program while pregnant, your recovery will be easier...I promise you...I can guarantee it! You will find that under that extra baby weight is an already toned body. Don't let this pregnancy pass you by! The time to get healthy is now...lets do it!

Training for Pregnancy

You know physical activity is not just safe, it is beneficial for mom and the baby, but the question is: what type of exercise is best during pregnancy? This was the question I set out to answer for myself. It is important to understand the physiological changes that occur to the female body while pregnant. You really are different. Most obviously you are growing enlarged breasts (to the delight of most) and growing an enlarged waistline (to the dislike of most) and maybe an enlarged ass (to the dislike of all). The first two changes will shift your center of gravity forward (the enlarged ass does not compensate). In terms of exercise, this puts you at potential risk of injury because you may misjudge your step or lose your balance. At the same time, it creates a unique training opportunity. It is this potential risk factor that I based my novel maternal training program on. If you are going to experience something that will make you less steady on your feet, why would you ignore it and thereby increase your theoretical risk of getting injured because of it? You could lose your balance going down a flight of stairs, right? Doesn't it make a lot more sense to work on improving your balance and stability early in your pregnancy so that by the time your center of gravity begins to change, your stabilizing muscles are so toned that you experience no loss of stability at all? Stability training is one element of the Mommy Fabulous Program.

Reinforcing joint strength by muscle toning is another element of the Mommy Fabulous Fitness Program. Pregnancy hormones have taken over your body and they are doing more than giving you that radiant glow. The hormone relaxin causes the joints in the pelvis to, well, relax so that the baby can pass through during delivery.[59] Unfortunately, all ligaments and joints become lax, not just the pelvis. This creates a theoretical risk for joint injury. Muscle toning exercises can mitigate the effects of joint laxity. To illustrate, when the ligaments in the hips became lax due to hormonal changes, toned strong hip muscles stabilize the joint, helping to protect it from injury. As pregnancy progresses, I encourage you to recognize your limitations and to exercise cautiously. This is not the ideal time for an inflexible person to practice doing the splits. But I feel it is a mistake to anticipate weaknesses and then play into them by doing nothing to address them. Another example is that the lower back becomes sore and aches when it becomes overstretched often due to poor posture, the added weight of the baby and the effects of relaxin on the spine. Nearly 75% of women experience back pain during pregnancy. Back pain can be minimized or completely avoided with the right exercises. By strengthening postural muscles, your back will be able to meet the challenge when it is taxed later in pregnancy.

Ligament laxity can cause the arches in the feet to flatten during pregnancy. Unlike other joints in the body that return to their normal pre-pregnancy position, the foot may not. Some women end up having to buy all new shoes because their foot is a larger size than before, or they now need to buy wide shoes. Some women develop flat feet during pregnancy which often require orthotic shoe inserts for the rest of their lives. You can help prevent this in two ways! First, it is very important to wear supportive footwear. Second, practicing balance, in early pregnancy in a safe and controlled way will strengthen the muscles of the foot resulting in improved arch support. It is important to stress *safe and controlled* here. No one wants to fall. An example would be standing on one foot, with the other just a few inches from the floor, with a sturdy chair to grab if you lose your balance. Try working up to 60 seconds on each foot. Balance training is an integral part of the Mommy Fabulous Program.

A mother is the center of the world's greatest balancing act.

For those of you who already have a child, you know what I mean. Baby in one arm, purse on shoulder, keys in your hand, bags in the other, closing the door with your foot…sounds dangerous! Until you are a mother, you don't understand the meaning of the words multitasking, juggling and balancing act. The Mommy Fabulous program will train you to catch the pacifier before it hits the floor, regain stability when you trip and balance all cumbersome items in your hands.

In general, women tend to have three physically weak areas: the core (abdominal muscles), the hips and the glutes (the butt muscles). Unfortunately the nature of pregnancy exacerbates these weaknesses. Pregnancy stretches out a weak waist, spreads weak hips and packs extra pounds in these three unfortunate places. The Mommy Fabulous Fitness Program targets those weak areas so that by the time you deliver, they are more toned than before. Looking fabulous postpartum isn't the only incentive to focus on the areas you either ignore, or haven't figured out how to target effectively. These weak spots tend to cause pregnancy related aches and pains in the second and third trimester.

Strong abs will save your back. This is true whether you are pregnant or not. People often experience back pain because they have poor core strength. Strengthening your abdominal muscles is important because the changing shape of your body is going to put additional stress on your back. Abdominal muscles maintain posture. Many of the exercises in this program are designed to strengthen your entire core while improving your posture.

Save Your Back Tips

If you stay in one position for a long time, your muscles get stiff. These muscles pull on the spine putting pressure on the discs. When spinal discs are stressed, this often results in an aching back. Move around every 30 minutes, and I don't just mean changing positions on the couch. Get up and walk to another room and back or do some stretches. This increases blood flow, loosens up the muscles and allows fluid to flow back into the spine, re-hydrating the discs. Never bend over to pick something up! Besides the fact that you probably do not want to draw attention to your increasingly large backside, lifting with your back strains the muscles, even if the object is light. When you pick up an object at arm's length by bending over, you are putting up to five times the amount of force on your spine than if you were to squat down and lift.

Strong abs can save themselves. Women with weak abs are at higher risk of developing diastasis recti. This is a painless separation of the abdominal muscles that occurs due to hormonal changes and the increasing physical stresses on the abdominal wall during pregnancy. When you are standing, the abdominal wall supports the uterus. The muscles of the abdomen must lengthen to accommodate your growing baby. Weak muscles may simply separate instead of being able to handle the tension. Women carrying multiple babies and very petite women are also at increased risk. Abdominal muscle separation can occur anytime in the last half of pregnancy. While the condition can be treated through physiotherapy postpartum, it will interfere with and prolong your abdominal recovery. Who wants to have to go through therapy after delivery? Another reason the Mommy Fabulous program focuses on the core is that during pregnancy the abs often get stretched to the point that the woman can not control or feel them anymore. When you lose touch with one of your body parts, it can be difficult to regain control of it. Postpartum it is VERY difficult to get a flat stomach (ever again) if you can not mentally control your abdominal muscles. It is very much like a newborn learning how to draw. Some may be quick to figure out how to use their mind to make their fingers do what they want, but most children between one and five are not great artists; and most moms don't have the stomach they want one to five years postpartum and some never figure out how to get control of their abs. The Mommy Fabulous program will ensure you maintain abdominal tone and control so that a gorgeous postpartum stomach is easily attainable.

When hip and butt muscles are weak, the hip and knee joints absorb all the impact of any activity, including something as simple as walking. This results in many overuse injuries such as tendonitis, strains down the backside, and bursitis. Add the extra weight and physical stress of a pregnancy and you are likely to feel an ache or two in these joints. You should not skip exercises for the hips or butt. Once your abdominal muscles are stretched to the point where you feel you can not control them well, your hips and glutes will be the stabilizing muscles that maintain your balance. If they are weak, your lower back will have to bear the entire burden.

Many pregnant women complain that their hips ache at night. At around the twentieth week of pregnancy, you should begin sleeping on your side. You may have trouble sleeping if this is not your usual position. In this new position, you will be lying on one hip, which will be supported by the bed, but the hip on top will be overly stretched because your knees are not as tall as your pelvis. This position can become painful for the hip joint during pregnancy, even if you are switching sides during the course of the night. During the third trimester turning over is not nearly as easy as it is now, and tossing just a few times during the night can cause you to lose precious sleep time. Strong hip muscles support the hip and take some of the strain off the joint. Strong hips don't ache, or at least ache much less than weak hips.

Side Sleeping Posture

You are going to need extra pillows. Get a body pillow (a luxury I didn't have, but wished I did) or one to two regular pillows to support your body. The first one should be placed between your knees. Elevate the knee of the top leg so that it is aligned with the hip joint. You will probably have to fold the pillow in half to get the height. The second pillow should be placed in one of two ways. It should either be lined up parallel in front of you as you lie on your side so you can place your belly on it. Or you can lie on top of it by lining the pillow up perpendicular with your waist and laying your belly on it. This keeps your spine aligned, and takes some of the belly weight off the lower back.

The Mommy Fabulous Workout Program is designed to do just that…make you look and feel fabulous after you deliver. Every exercise is specifically designed to meet the demands of pregnancy and motherhood and to target commonly weak, unshapely or ignored areas of the female body for all fitness levels. These exercises will be challenging and at the same time be safe. Technique is important to the effectiveness and safety of these exercises. The following two chapters explore common technique rules that can be applied to most all exercises, activities and daily life.

Chapter 11

Techniques That Make Exercise More Effective

If you workout smart, you will find that it is easier to stay fit than you thought. When you workout using the Mommy Fabulous method you will find that you can fatigue your muscles without slaving. And it is fun! The Mommy Fabulous method encompasses four fundamental elements that need to be practiced during every exercise. These elements will make any exercise more effective. Practice these while you exercise and you will see and feel results faster.

Control

Most people lift a weight too quickly (momentum), pause at the top (resting) and let the weight fall back to the starting position (gravity). At least 50% of this technique is passive, and therefore not effective. Muscle strength develops during contraction *and* when the muscle is stretched while under tension. This is the *return to starting* part of an exercise; the part most people let gravity or momentum do. Mommy Fabulous focuses equally on the accent and the decent of a rep. At this point, you have less than nine months to increase your muscle to fat ratio (which will increase your metabolism) so every minute you exercise should be maximized. This means controlling the entire range of an exercise. You should have 100% control over the weight, gravity and your muscles 100% of the time. Momentum should play no role in these exercises. During a biceps curl you should feel the muscle contracting as you bring the weight up, squeezing at the top and stretching as the weight is lowered. You should practice control during cardio exercises as well. When you do a jumping jack, you should not be flinging your arms over your head and letting gravity drop them back. Intentionally use the arm muscles to move the arms. Controlling your muscles burns more calories and produces better results.

Abdominal Visualization

During any given exercise, your abdominal muscles should be engaged. Mommy Fabulous is one of few fitness methods that actualize the term *core*. It is called *the core* for a reason. Mommy Fabulous makes your core the center of every exercise. Contracting your core, by pulling your belly button toward your spine and holding it there through the entirety of the exercise is a critical element of every exercise in this book. This core contraction technique is very challenging. As you are doing a biceps curl, you won't even notice you have *let go* of your abs. To master this technique, you must understand how to engage your core. Refer to the pictures on the following page. Notice how a flexed rectus abdominus looks different than a flexed transverse abdominus. After doing this program you will be so in-tune with your abs that you will be able to control these different muscles and flex them independently. Doing traditional sit ups and crunches will not give you core strength; they target the wrong muscles. It is the muscles underneath the external trunk that make the abdomen flat. The core muscles function to control and limit movement of the torso. Think of the rectus abdominus like a corset. When contracted, your torso can not move much. So if you are moving during a sit up, you can see that the core can not be working.

Anatomy Lesson

External Trunk Muscles

Rectus Abdominus Contracted

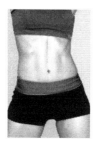

External Oblique Contracted

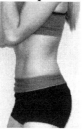

External Trunk: You have muscles that run from your rib cage to your pelvis called the rectus abdominus. These make a six pack when developed. On each side of the rectus abdominus there are muscles called the obloquies. The obliques wrap around from your back, to the front of your pelvis. When developed these muscles pull everything in giving you a small waist. The rectus abdominus, the external obliques and the erector spinal muscle (lower back) make up the external trunk muscles that are responsible for movement.

Core Muscle

Transverse Abdominus Contracted

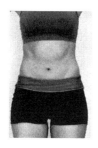

Core Muscles: Underneath the external trunk muscles are deep core muscles. The core muscles function to provide spinal stabilization and assist with breathing. The core is made up of the diaphragm, pelvic floor, transversospinalis and the transverse abdominus. The transverse abdominus is our main target muscle, this where people get the pooch tummy below the belly button. When developed, these are the muscles that make your stomach flat. You need to learn how to engage the transverse abdominus. It will be challenging because the core muscles are often weak and underused. Learn to control the transverse abdominus while pregnant and you will have a flat stomach after birth in no time!

Try to control your rectus abdominus by drawing your belly button to your spine. Do not suck in your stomach to cave the belly button inward by inhaling; this is using your lungs and diaphragm (a core muscle, but the wrong one). Rather, you are contracting a muscle, so you should be blowing out as you pull the transverse abdominus tight and back toward your spine. Because you are contracting the transverse abdominus independently from the diaphragm, you should be able to inhale and exhale while keeping it contracted. It is a deep muscle that is often weak. If you are having trouble locating the transverse abdominus, lay down on your back with your knees bent and feet flat on the floor. Try to curl your pubic bone up toward your chin without using your butt muscles. You will notice the transverse abdominus pulls the stomach back toward the spine. This is called a Pelvic Tilt; refer to page 103 for more help.

As a pregnant woman, you have a visualization reminder to keep your core engaged while exercising- your baby. As you draw your navel to your spine, imagine your core muscles wrapped tightly around your baby. Imagine your abs as arms cradling your baby. Keep your abs engaged during the entire length of an exercise by remembering to not let your abs *drop* the baby. The core muscles respond best to abdominal exercises with small ranges of motion or positions with no torso motion held for a period of time.

As you are working on Mommy Fabulous balance challengers visualize that only your baby exists. Your baby (and transverse abdominus) is the center of your stability. Focus on the baby, focus on your abs. The harder you contract your core, the greater balance you will have. The harder you contract your core and focus on the baby, you will notice that your arms and legs exist less with regards to balance. Try it. Stand on one leg, draw your core in and imagine the baby is the only thing that exists. The more you try to balance with your arms, the more distracted you will be and the less control you will have over your ab muscles. This is a very good bonding exercise. Each time you contract your abdomen, think of it as hugging your baby. Focus on the communication of love with your baby as you do a crunch. Imagine your baby snuggled in your womb getting a little hug with each rep. Make sure you are pulling your baby inward for the hug/crunch and not pushing your core outward and your baby away from your spine.

Skin Bonus

If you keep your abs strong, your waistline will increase more slowly over the course of your pregnancy. This allows your skin time to stretch gradually. You may feel like strong abs are holding your baby back. Don't worry; there is plenty of room in your abdomen for your tiny baby with no change in your waistline. When your baby needs more room, even the strongest abs in the world couldn't hold a baby back. Plus you won't have to buy as many pregnancy clothes. Save that money for a new postpartum Mommy Fabulous wardrobe!

Concentration

Concentration is not an automatic ability. Many people go through life on autopilot. Have you ever arrived somewhere and couldn't remember the drive over? Pregnancy is the perfect time to practice concentration. You will find it easier to become in-tune with your body because you will have a heightened awareness.

Maintaining proper form while exercising takes great concentration. Proper form is especially important while pregnant because it helps prevent injury. It is easy to get lost in music, start thinking about what still fits or what you will have for dinner. Your workout is not the time for daydreaming, save that for when you are at work. I am sure you will concentrate on breathing and working through a contraction while taking a birthing class, so focus while you workout because working out is labor prep too!

Not everyone has great concentration, but this is something that can be practiced. I find weightlifting very meditative. You must concentrate on the muscle the exercise is isolating, your posture, your abs, your breathing and controlling and coordinating all of those to produce a smooth motion. It is mentally challenging and fun. It is the ultimate stress reliever because you have no time to think about other things when you are so focused. During labor, pain will get your attention. People often respond to pain with fear and panic. If you practice concentrating on muscle contraction for nine months, you will be less likely to fall into the panic-fear cycle when you are in labor. You will be very used to muscle contractions and how to work through them. You will be able to concentrate despite distraction. Some women use concentration as a pain coping mechanism. If you can focus on something else, the pain doesn't feel as bad.

Breathing

Breathing is the forth essential element of Mommy Fabulous. Slow, deliberate breathing will help you maintain control and concentration. As a general rule, breathe out during the hard part of the exercise and breathe in during the easier part. The natural tendency is to hold your breath during a muscle contraction. During a workout and during labor, holding your breath during a contraction will deprive your muscles of oxygen they need to contract and will result in fatigue and cramping. Poor breathing will sabotage you. Proper breathing will improve your performance.

As your muscles begin to fatigue during an exercise you naturally want to speed up the reps to be finished. That is, people tend to start out slow and controlled and finish at a much faster tempo. However, your body doesn't usually increase your breathing rate to finish quickly. If you are lifting with each exhale, your breathing should keep your pace slow and even. As you focus on breathing with contraction, your mind will be less likely to wonder and you will be more able to maintain proper form.

Normally, people tend to breathe a bit shallowly. The ribs extend a bit as we inhale and collapse as we exhale. The breathing technique I recommend conditions your lungs for labor. It will also decrease breathlessness when doing normal activities such as climbing a few stairs during the second and third trimester. Breathe deeply. As you slowly inhale the diaphragm lowers, increasing the pressure in your abdominal cavity. Your rib cage will expand and slightly elevate. Do not allow your shoulders to shrug upwards or your back muscles to tighten upwards. Actively pull your shoulder blades downward. As you inhale deeply fully filling the lungs with oxygen your abdomen should expand outward. Normally we exhale passively by just collapsing the diaphragm, but exhalation can be controlled. Draw your naval inward, toward your spine by contracting the transverse abdominus. The pressure created while contracting the core will push the air out. This breathing technique can be a workout it's self!

Diaphragmatic Breathing

Sit down on the ground with the legs crossed or sit in a chair. Place the right hand on the middle of your chest and the left hand over your belly button. Inhale and feel your chest expand and elevate with your right hand. Continue to inhale and feel your abdomen expand under your left hand. Then pull your abs in toward your spine and feel how this pushes the air out of your mouth. Continue to pull the abs in until the lunges are nearly empty and repeat.

If you have not practiced this technique before, it may take awhile to get the hang of it. Make sure you get the breathing down before adding an exercise to it. Practice this technique while driving, sitting on the toilet and during stretching. Remember, exhalation should occur during the contraction part of an exercise and inhalation should occur while a muscle is being stretched. Diaphragmatic breathing uses core muscles, so mastering this technique will increase your stability as well as increase the safety and effectiveness of any exercise. When you are performing resistance training, do not empty the lungs completely when you exhale. Do not hold your breath at any point and do not purse your lips together as you exhale. Forcefully exhaling through pursed lips should not be practiced while pregnant because it can increase blood pressure.

Common Mistakes that Decrease Effectiveness

You are spending the time in the gym; you might as well get all the benefits from it. In order to workout safely and effectively you must choose to do activities at the appropriate speed, select the appropriate amount of weight and perform an exercise at an appropriate intensity.

- Speed or tempo: This is an exercise element that can be varied. The perfect speed that a repetition should be done at is the speed where you have 100% control over the weight. Many people perform weightlifting too fast, and end up swinging the weights more than lifting them. Due to the increased safety concern for the pregnant body, as well as the necessity to maintain proper posture, I recommend that each rep be approximately eight seconds long. From the starting position, it should take four seconds to reach the execution position, and four seconds to return to the starting position. An eight second rep will also ensure that you inhale deeply and exhale likewise. I do not recommend pausing between reps or during a rep when you switch the direction. People tend to overestimate the pause time and use the time to rest the muscle rather than keeping it under tension.

- Too much weight: This is the most common mistake people make. When you choose too much weight, you risk injury, but that is not the only downside. When using a weight that is too heavy, you compensate by using other muscle groups to do the work the target muscle is too weak to do. This usually disrupts proper posture which is essential during pregnancy. Don't underestimate the work you can do with your own body weight and gravity.

Your Body Weight May Be Enough

Assuming you have no significant medical issues, the weight of your leg is approximately 9-10% of the weight of your entire body. So if you weigh 140 pounds, then your leg weighs about 14 pounds. As your pregnancy progresses and you gain weight, your leg will also become heavier. If you begin doing leg lifts with a 14 pound leg, and gain 30 pounds during pregnancy, you will be doing leg lifts with a 17 pound leg at the end. The same exercises will be more challenging simply because of your situation. Your arm is approximately 6.5% of your body weight.[60] If a woman weighs 140 pounds, her arm weighs about nine pounds. If you are doing lateral shoulder raises and you swing your arms up and down like a bird, your shoulders are not even getting a nine pound benefit.

- Using momentum and gravity: Most people perform exercises incorrectly by using momentum and gravity to do the work, so the weight of the dumbbell doesn't really even count. They may choose a ten pound dumbbell (too heavy for shoulder muscles), but because they are using momentum to swing the arm upwards they are not isolating the shoulder muscle. They are only getting a fraction of work out of the exercise. On the way down, people often let gravity return the weight to starting. You should have 100% control over the weight at all times. Because you will be following proper technique, your nine pound arm may be all the resistance you need. Holding no weight, you will be getting a more effective workout than you would if you were swinging a ten pound dumbbell around.

- Doing the wrong exercises: Many people choose the wrong exercises for their goals. It is difficult for a person with no formal training to know what exercises are the right ones for them. Good exercises, performed correctly, will *not* give you the results you want, if they were designed to accomplish a different goal. Even fit people who workout regularly may be doing exercises that are not in their best interest. Poor exercise selection will not be a problem for you because this program was designed to challenge and develop specific needs of the changing pregnant body while maximizing safety and effectiveness. These exercises were also specifically chosen because they will shorten the amount of time it will take you to look fabulous postpartum.

Guidelines for Choosing Exercises on Your Own

Mommy Fabulous is a balanced full-body program. After flipping through Chapter 14, you may notice that some classic gym exercises are not included in this program. You may want to select additional exercises to add to your repertoire, but how will you know if they are appropriate?

1. Generally, avoid exercises where you are bent over, which will strain your back. Rowing and deadlifts strain the lower back; now is not the time.
2. I did not include many exercises done on machines because a machine is locked into a specific range of motion and is designed for a specific body size (usually a man's). A pregnant body is changing and a machine doesn't allow for enough adjustment. Machines can also put unnatural forces on the body. For example, certain calf raise machines put too much downward force on the pregnant spine, as do squat machines and shoulder shrug machines. You also miss out on the core benefits of standing exercises. Cable machine exercises are your best bet.
3. I don't recommend exercises that involve twisting or trunk rotation if you are a beginner at weightlifting or exercise in general. An experienced lifter should phase out twisting and rotation no later than week 25 on. Use your judgment here, once you feel like your growing belly is affecting your spinal range of motion, don't push it. Rotational movement results in a lot of muscle compensation when the spine is immobile. There are plenty of exercises that effectively train your body without the strain torso rotation puts on the small muscle fibers of your back.
4. Don't perform compound exercises. A compound exercise combines two movements, like a reverse lunge and then a forward high knee. During pregnancy compound moves are discouraged for safety reasons. There is back stress during the transition between the two moves. When you transition from your weight bearing forward as you lunge back, to weight bearing back as you do a forward high knee, the lower back has to compensate. During pregnancy your back is going to be taxed enough without doing exercises that make it vulnerable to strain. High knees are great, reverse lunges are great, do them separately. As a trainer I usually discourage compound movements, even for those who are not pregnant. When done as a compound movement, people tend to do a squat with poor alignment and a sloppy bicep curl. They don't get the full benefit of either exercise and the back usually bears the brunt of the work when one or the other set of muscles gets tired.
5. Keep exercises where you sit to a minimum. The core has to work harder when you are standing and balancing. Sitting also decreases the number of calories burned.
6. It is safer for your back to perform exercises where both arms complete the movement together rather than alternating (rowing, lateral shoulder raises, bicep curls, etc.). Alternating legs is fine.
7. During the second and third trimesters, you will want to avoid prolonged periods of bouncing, as in trampolines or jumping rope. This will overstretch the pelvic floor as it has to absorb all the downward force of your baby with each bounce. Aerobic classes can be continued with low-impact modifications; most moves can be performed without jumping.
8. During the second and third trimesters you will want to be cautious of activities that require sudden changes in direction or quick changes in speed. This is where joint laxity can do more than theoretical joint injury. This includes wind sprints or cardio drills.

The Mommy Fabulous method was designed for a pregnant woman by a pregnant woman- me! It is designed to help you workout with confidence, knowing that what you are doing is safe and beneficial. In the best case scenario, you will have a workout buddy who helps you maintain form and hands you weights. If you are working out alone, that is fine too. Just make sure you use extra caution when getting into the starting positions.

I don't think I should lift weights because I don't want to get bulky.

This is unlikely to happen for a number of reasons. First, muscle mass or bulk, is stimulated by testosterone. Women have 30% less testosterone than the average man, so it is much more difficult to put on bulk the way a man can. Additionally, there is a lot more to putting on bulk than you may realize. Bodybuilders, both professional and hobby builders, do their homework. There is a whole field of science involved in technique, program design and periodization schedules. The ability to build bulk has a lot to do with diet and supplements. Bodybuilders spend a lot of time at the gym. I highly doubt that you will accidentally workout like a bodybuilder and accidentally build bulk. While you are pregnant you should not be lifting weights heavy enough that would lead to bulk anyway. This program is designed to create a lean, tight postpartum body.

I have lifted weights in the past and tend to put on muscle mass quickly.

Still, I have many women who, even after hearing me explain the above, say that they have this certain body type that builds muscle very quickly and they usually have a story about how they worked out one time for a month and gained weight, or their pants got tight because their thighs got bigger. (Coincidently it is never men who have this problem; they seem to have to work hard for bulk.) There are two reasons this can happen. When you exercise, you are hungrier. People generally have a body area they want to fix, and it is usually this area that their body tends to store new pounds. If a woman who is interested in slimming her thighs begins working out and eating more than she is burning off, it is likely that the extra calories she is consuming are being stored on her thighs. However, she has not noticed she has started eating more and her fears are confirmed, doing squats has resulted in bulkier thighs. Then, when she stops working out, she also consumes less calories, and therefore is able to shed the thigh thickness. In her mind, this again proves that it was the resistance training that caused the increased thigh circumference. Toned, tight muscles take up less room than flabby, soft, unshapely muscles. I have worked up to bench pressing 100 pounds, and I am a size two. I am strong, but I am in no way bulky.

The second reason for this illusion is body shape. If you have a wide waist and no hips, working your hips might make your hips wider. This may not sound good, but it will create an hourglass figure. Wouldn't you rather have an hourglass shape? There are many different body shapes that wear the same size. Your clothes may start feeling tight but a different style in the same size may fit perfectly. Overall you will look better. Likewise, if you are too thin for your frame, the body may respond to the activity and caloric intake more quickly. When women get too thin, they lose their curves. It is possible you have been too thin for a long time, maybe even since adolescence. Nobody likes to think they are gaining weight, or that their clothes are getting tighter, but you may look hotter as a size six than as a size four. Would you rather have a tight lifted butt and slender curvy hips that require a size six pants or a flabby butt and cellulite thighs that fit into a pair of size four jeans? The beauty of weightlifting during pregnancy is that you will be growing out of your cloths no matter what, so you will not be able to blame it on physical fitness. Trust me; with this workout you will shed those extra pounds after you deliver revealing a tight butt, curvy hips, small waist and slender thighs.

Chapter 12

Body English

When you hear the word *posture* you probably think, stand up straight. Posture is a lot more than standing erect with the shoulders pulled back. Posture principals can be applied to any position or activity you are engaged in. Poor posture is often what limits people physically, causes fatigue and is responsible for most daily aches and pains. The following body alignment rules will make work, daily life and exercises safer and more effective. Don't sabotage your workouts with these simple Body English mistakes.

1. Head alignment: When the going gets tough, people often put their head down to meet the challenge. Sounds like a winning move, but it's a big mistake. Instead, face your physical challenge head on; meaning always keep your neck aligned with the spine. When you curl your neck down, you are straining the muscles of your neck and back. When these muscles get tight you will end up more sore than if you had performed an exercise correctly. Many people drop their heads to read or type as well. Look with your eyes, not with your head!

2. Wrist alignment: When lifting weights, keep wrists straight. Don't curl the wrist forward at the top of a bicep curl and don't bend the wrist backward when doing a bench press. When your wrist is at an angle to your forearm, it takes tension off the muscles and places it on the wrist joint and ligaments. Poor wrist alignment is the cause of carpel tunnel syndrome.

3. Soft joints: For most exercises, joints should not be locked straight, but rather have a slight bend (with the exception of the wrist). Good posture means that the knees and hips should be slightly bent, or *soft*. When you are extending your arms or legs during a rep, you should never extend the joint to a completely straight position; there should always be a slight bend.

4. Placing hands on the hips: This tips the pelvis forward, pointing the tailbone back and out, messing up your spinal alignment and preventing you from contracting the core muscles. A pelvis tipped forward encourages the lower back muscles to contract to stabilize the body. Proper posture means the tailbone should be pointed downward to protect the back. The tailbone should be directed downward by contracting the core. However, you can not activate your core if your hands are on your hips tipping your pelvis forward. The core should be the center of every exercise. It is a common mistake for people to put their hands on their hips when doing lunges, kicks, calf raises or high knees. Keep your hands in fists next to your chin as a boxer, or together as if praying. During the day, if you must put your hands on your hips, rotate your wrists so that the thumb is on the front side of your pelvis tipping it backward into proper alignment.

5. Bending the ankles: While performing any activity, a squat, getting into a car, getting off the couch or picking something up, your knees should never move forward past your toes. If you are standing, and bend only your knees, your whole body would fall backwards. Therefore, the ankles must bend in coordination with the knees do to prevent falling. The problem is that most

people over-bend their ankles as they bend their knees, so that the knee joint moves forward past the toes. This puts a lot of stress on the knee joint and does not challenge the leg muscles as much it should. Ankles should always be underneath the knees, not behind them. During pregnancy you are going to get heavier. This is an opportunity to develop your leg muscles, not to wear down the cartilage in the knee joint. Practice this alignment your whole life to save knee mobility into old age.

6. Spinal Alignment: Maintaining good posture generally means that you are standing with feet shoulder width apart, toes pointed forward. Weight should be distributed equally on each foot and equally between the balls and the heels of each foot. The hip bones should be pointed forward and the shoulders should line up with the hips (no rotation at the waist). Shoulders should be pulled back and down with chest lifted. There should be a natural curve in the lower back. Abs should be engaged so that the tailbone is pointed downward.

Alignment will become increasingly important as your body changes during pregnancy. A good pelvic tilt or core contraction usually corrects body alignment. With proper posture, you can safely perform most physical activities. It is usually not an activity that is risky during pregnancy, but rather poor form when doing an activity that creates potential risk. Read the examples below that demonstrate how Body English determines how effective an exercise is.

Body English at the Gym

High Knee Exercise

Refer to page 113, the High Knee. Get into the starting position. Now that you are here, I want you to understand that the exercise looks like body movement, but it is not. The back, torso, head and arms should not move. At the same time, the foot, ankle and knee joint should not change position. The hip muscle and hip bone alignment should not change either. You may be thinking, *how can I move the lower half of my body if I am not supposed to be moving anything?* The only thing that should move is the quadriceps thigh muscle. You should control the muscle to elongate or stretch which will lower the leg, and you will contract or shorten the length of the muscle which will cause the leg to rise. Contraction or relaxation of the quadriceps thigh muscle will cause the joint angle between the leg and the pelvis to become smaller or larger. You should focus on how the muscle will change the angle of the joint, not on how changing the joint angle will change the position of the leg. It may sound like the exact same thing, but it is not. If you change the joint angle to change the leg position, then you will use mostly gravity and momentum to move the leg.

Stair Stepper

Poor posture decreases the effectiveness of any activity and strains joints, ligaments and muscle groups. When you start leaning forwards or backwards during any activity, your body is trying to compensate because your postural muscles are tired. To illustrate, when a person is on a stair climber and they are getting tired, you will often see them leaning on the machine, or trying to support their body weight on the machine. By doing this, the person is straining their lower back and neck, placing excessive tension on their wrists and shoulders and taking pressure off their leg muscles by supporting their weight elsewhere. It is much better to simply take the intensity down, by decreasing speed or switching to an easier program and maintaining proper form. With regards to weightlifting, stop when your muscles are too fatigued to maintain proper posture. Getting in a few extra reps with poor form is more likely to leave you with a back muscle strain than produce a noticeable benefit.

Body English in Everyday Life

Many injuries occur due to poor Body English during everyday activities. People usually strain their back reaching for the bottle of shampoo not when they are lifting a dumbbell. The Body English concept is to understand what muscles perform a given movement and to align your body so that other muscle groups don't overcompensate.

Picking Something Up Off the Floor

Don't strain your back bending over to pick something up! Your back is going to be working overtime during pregnancy, and it doesn't need the stress of lifting your torso and the baby hanging off the front of it, plus whatever it is you are picking up. All lifting should be done as a squat. Squat lifting can, and should, be started at the beginning of pregnancy to develop the quadriceps or thigh muscles. During late pregnancy the squat can still be performed by angling the legs outward at the hip to make room between your knees for the baby. The squat should be performed by pushing the hips and butt backwards, as if you were going to sit down. The knees should not travel forward extending over the toes. Feet should remain flat on the ground. You should pick up the item using your arms (bicep curl) to bring it closer to your body, rather than rocking your body forward onto the balls of your feet and using your back. As you stand up, press all your weight through your heels and stand up straight. To maintain proper back alignment, it can help to look up at the ceiling as you are standing up.

Picking Something Up Off a Counter

Apply exercise principles while doing everyday tasks like getting milk out of the refrigerator. Most people just grab the milk carton without thinking about it. Doing a proper biceps curl involves intentional bicep contraction, body alignment, coordinated breathing and core activation. Both mindless and intentional lifting may look like the same movement, but when you grab the milk, you usually use your back to bring it closer to you, you do a body alignment change to heave (using many muscles rather than the bicep alone) and then use momentum to bring it to the counter and gravity to set it down. Very little work has been done by the bicep muscle, or any muscle for that matter. Learning to control your muscles will result in you having more effective and shorter workouts for the rest of your life while looking more toned and fabulous.

Chapter 13

Your Personalized Exercise Program

It is important to keep a well rounded workout routine, especially while pregnant. Child birth requires many different types of physical elements from stamina and endurance to respiratory conditioning, to muscle contraction strength to pain management. And being flexible really helps as well. Pregnancy taxes the lower back and requires more lower body strength while motherhood requires more upper body and upper back strength. The Mommy Fabulous program will address all of these needs.

How do you measure up today?

Current physical activity recommendations for adults include cardio or aerobic exercise as well as resistance, strength-building, and weight-bearing activities. According to the President's Council for Physical Fitness and Sports, the following is the minimal amount of activity an average healthy person needs to maintain a minimal overall level of fitness.[61]

Activity	Time Requirement		Example
Cardio	20 continuous minutes	3 days per week	jogging, swimming, cycling, aerobics
Strenghth	20 minutes	2 days per week	weightlifting
Muscle Endurance	30 minutes	3 days per week	balance training, calisthenics, resistance training
Flexibility	10-12 minutes	7 days per week	stretching, yoga

This amounts to five days of weight training, three days of cardio and stretching everyday for a minimum of 40-50 minutes of activity seven days a week. This is the minimum amount you need! If you already exercise everyday- congratulations! You are already on your way to being Mommy Fabulous-but you need to keep it up over the next nine months. If you don't get this much activity in a normal day...you need to. Now is the best time to increase your activity level. The American College of Obstetrics and Gynecology agrees. The ACOG recommends that "If you are active now, pregnancy need not cause you to alter your fitness routine." The ACOG also advises, "If you have not been active, now is a good time to start."[14]

Pregnancy provides an opportunity to try other forms of exercise which, you will later find, will strengthen neglected aspects of your fitness and abilities. A pregnant person should not start training for a marathon, or a century ride, or start power lifting. But the truth is that every pregnant woman will need to modify their training regimen to accommodate their changing abilities and many pregnant women will find themselves taking up new activities. Even those Olympic athletes among us can not continue to high jump or pole vault while pregnant and you can not continue to scuba dive or play contact sports. For those of you who do not workout regularly, this is the perfect time to start lifting light weights, cycling or jumping into a pool. The luxury is that you are pregnant, so you don't have to be self conscious that you can only lift two pound dumbbells or swim 25 yards and need a break.

Your first trimester is sort of a free-be exercise-wise because there is no need to modify your training program if you worked out before you became pregnant with the exceptions noted in Chapter 4. Continue to enjoy non-contact sports, running, jumping or vigorous cardio. The more physically fit you are able to stay in your first trimester, the easier your third will be. Even though you don't necessarily have to change your fitness routine in the first trimester, it is important that you incorporate the Mommy Fabulous exercises into your routine now, rather than waiting. By the time you decide to switch gears you may not be conditioned to this type of exercise.

The Mommy Fabulous Fitness Program focuses on weight bearing, resistance and strength building exercises. If you already lift weights, I recommend reading the exercise descriptions in Chapter 14 because I give body alignment suggestions that protect the pregnant body and make the exercises you already do more effective. Add in exercises from Chapter 14 to work muscle groups in a new way and focus on preparing your body for the second and third trimester. Please refer to Chapter 11 and 12 for appropriate form, which is important while pregnant because you do not want to strain your muscles when you need them most. I can not express how important weightlifting is for women and that includes pregnant women.

Most people believe that the key to looking great postpartum is just losing the weight. A woman can be a skinny size four and still be flabby or have cellulite. Weight bearing and weightlifting exercises make these regions firmer. For the pregnant woman, weightlifting is a great way to exercise because it is low impact and works the heart as well as the muscles. Weightlifting increases the muscle to fat ratio in the body which raises a person's metabolism. A higher metabolism means more calories are burned at rest. Think of it this way: Two people are sitting on the couch watching TV. One lifts weights at the gym and the other person always does cardio on the treadmill. The person who lifts weights can burn more calories while sitting on the couch watching TV than the person who does cardio because their metabolisms are working at different rates. How cool is that? During pregnancy this will become very important for weight management. Women who rely on cardio often end up gaining too much weight, because their cardio abilities are drastically reduced as pregnancy progresses. Without a strong muscle based metabolism and weightlifting program for exercise, they aren't able to burn enough calories to keep up with their eating. If time is a factor, you are better off focusing on weights. If you can develop and maintain a solid metabolism while pregnant by building muscle, when you deliver your baby, you won't have to get back in shape. Getting back in shape is HARD. It is way easier to stay in shape than to try to climb up the fitness ladder. And I feel it is way easier to get in shape during the first six months of pregnancy than the first six months of motherhood. After delivery you may be sleep deprived, you will have less time, and your body will be more fragile at two weeks postpartum than two weeks pregnant. If you maintain a good metabolism, the pounds will melt off after the baby is born. I know…having pounds melt away sounds like a gimmick, but I can explain. If you develop a stronger metabolism while pregnant by building muscle, then you will continue to have a high metabolism after you deliver, provided you stay active. The difference is that while pregnant you are eating extra calories to gain proper weight, after you deliver, you won't eat as many calories because the baby will not be consuming them. So your metabolism will still be strong, but you won't be eating as much…this means easier weight loss. Additionally, when you return to the gym you will be surprised that the exact training regimen you did the week before you went into labor is much easier. You will probably be ten pounds lighter without the baby and placenta. So the same exercises will be do-able and this will be motivating.

Pregnancy is weightlifting. Go to the gym and pick up two 15 pound dumbbells, one in each hand. Then I want you to cruise around the perimeter of the gym with them. How do your calves feel? How do your thighs feel? If this wore you out, get ready, because you will be weighing about thirty pounds more by the end of your pregnancy if not more. Every step you take, every day, will be like that lap around the gym. Are you ready? You have got time to develop muscle strength now!

Childbirth is weightlifting. Most women focus on cardio, but labor is not a cardio workout. Your heart rate doesn't get elevated much. Cardio will help with endurance during labor, but weightlifting will help with breathing through contractions. It will prepare you to mentally focus on muscle contraction despite pain and give you muscle control during a contraction.

Motherhood is weightlifting. Bend your elbows and face your palms to the ceiling as if you were a waiter carrying a tray. Now set a ten pound dumbbell on top of them. Stand there for two minutes. Your arms will begin to burn, you will try to adjust your posture to bear the load and your neck will begin to strain. The average newborn weighs seven pounds five ounces. Babies generally like to be held longer than two minutes a day. Now put a three pound diaper bag on one shoulder and the weight of the car seat carrier with baby inside in the other hand. Heavy? Are you ready? Weightlifting will prepare you to lift properly, posture properly and keep you from developing aches and pains. The time to develop muscle strength is now!

Making Your Workout Plan

As a general rule, plan your workouts so you avoid consecutive days of hard exercise. You also want to avoid working the same muscle group on consecutive days. If you do a cycling class on Tuesday, don't do leg exercises on Monday or Wednesday. Abdominals are the only muscle group that can and should be worked daily. Each workout should begin with a warm-up and end with a cool-down, both averaging about five to ten minutes. The following workout schedules are designed for a healthy, low risk, singleton pregnancy. Find your fitness level below, beginner, intermediate, or advanced and follow the sample regimen to the best of your ability. These are just suggestions, use your own judgment and listen to your body. Every pregnancy progresses differently, so you will have to modify your schedule accordingly over time. If you have, or develop health issues, ask your doctor how they should affect your fitness routine and make appropriate adjustments. The most important thing when making a fitness schedule is that you make a plan that you can commit to.

Sample Workout Regimens
for a healthy, low risk, singleton pregnancy

Beginners
- **Fitness beginners** would be anyone who does not have a set workout schedule.
- Someone who is active in that they walk the dog.
- Someone who does not exercise at all; sedentary.

For women who have previously been sedentary, activities such as walking, swimming or stationary cycling pose the least risk of injury. Because of the theoretical risk of injury to joints, you should not start running or jogging. Many of the weightlifting exercises in this book can be safe and effective for you if you choose an appropriate weight. Two or three pound dumbbells should be used in most cases. For any bar exercises, use a 9 to 15 pound weighted bar or a closet dowel. Some of the exercises require no weight at all. A daily 30-minute exercise session is reasonable. Water aerobics and senior fitness classes may be a good choice for beginners. Below is a suggested schedule for a beginner; it follows the recommendations of the President's Council for Physical Fitness and Sports for the minimum amount of activity for a healthy person. If you feel you are capable of more, please be as active as you can be. Without medical complications, there is no reason to take your fitness down a notch.

Can I break my daily 30 minutes of activity into 10 minute sessions?
Some sources advise beginners to do this, but I personally feel it is ridiculous for a healthy person to do this. Instead of seven exercise sessions per week you are would be doing twenty-one! You

are more likely to complete one thirty minute session than keep up with three per day. You will also get more health benefits out of a solid thirty minute session. This is because you have a better chance of fatiguing a given muscle group when worked continuously. If you get into a pool and kick for ten minutes and then take a four hour break and repeat, your leg muscles will not have to work as hard and you will not build as much muscle. Building muscle means building a better metabolism. If thirty minutes seems daunting, remember that it is not a thirty minute all out sprint and you don't have to do one activity the whole time. Exercise can be performed at a comfortable intensity; refer to Chapter 9, the Perceived Exertion section. You can do ten minutes on a bike, ten minutes on an elliptical and ten minutes on a treadmill. My grossly obese clients can handle thirty minute sessions. It mostly comes down to motivation and desire.

Fitness Beginner
Suggested First Trimester Regimen

First, consider what activities you enjoy and what will keep you interested. You NEED to keep this up for nine months (and really for a lifetime). You are worth it and you will benefit from it during pregnancy, during labor and afterward.

1. Join a class or start a walking group
   - A low impact cardio class like spinning may be appropriate because you can pace yourself so it can be lower in intensity…sit in the back and don't worry about keeping up with the instructor. If you have been sedentary, classes for seniors and water aerobics are often a good choice for a pregnant woman because they are designed for people with limited mobility and are low in intensity.
   - If classes are not your thing, do two half hour cardio sessions per week
     - Great activities include speed walking (at least three miles per hour), bike riding or swimming.
2. Start weightlifting using the Easier Modifications of the Mommy Fabulous fitness techniques described in this book three to four times per week.
   - Do these exercises in the gym or at home in front of a mirror. A mirror will help you self-correct form and posture. You may want to practice without weights until you get the motions down.
   - If you feel you are getting stronger during the first half of your pregnancy and want to challenge yourself, add more exercises per muscle or try some Intermediate or Advanced Modifications, rather than trying heavier dumbbells.
3. Stretching: two 30 minute sessions per week
   - Stretching is important to reduce muscle soreness and keep your body limber. Stretching should occur before and after every aerobic activity. You can work some stretches in between weightlifting sets, but also dedicate a solid 30 minutes to stretching twice a week.
   - A prenatal yoga class might be a good option.
4. Abdominals: two 15 minute sessions per week
   - Ideally, abdominals should be challenged everyday. Keep abs engaged while doing aerobic activity. The Mommy Fabulous exercises are all core focused. A good strategy may be to add three sets of ten, of any ab exercise at the end of each workout. At the very least, do two 15 minute sessions of abdominals every week.

Here is how it might look:

Sample Workout Regimen for the Fitness Beginner During the First Trimester

Day	Activity	Length of Time
Monday	Water Aerobics or Stationary Bike	1hr or 30 minutes
Tuesday	Weightlifting Abs	30 minutes 15 minutes
Wednesday	Stretch Session	30 minutes
Thursday	Weightlifting	30 minutes
Friday	Walking or Swimming	30 minutes
Saturday	Abs Weightlifting	15 minutes 20 minutes
Sunday	Stretch Session or Prenatal Yoga	30 minutes or 1 hr

Sample Beginner Weightlifting Breakdown

Day	Muscle Groups	Frequency	
Tuesday	Biceps	1 exercise	3 sets of 8 reps
	Butt & Thighs	3 exercises	2 sets of 8 reps
	Abs	5 exercises	1 set each to fatigue
Thursday	Chest	1 exercise	3 sets of 8 reps
	Shoulders	1 exercise	3 sets of 8 reps
	Hips	2 exercises	3 sets of 8 reps
Saturday	Triceps	1 exercise	3 sets of 8 reps
	Back	1 exercise	3 sets of 8 reps
	Calves	1 exercise	3 sets of 8 reps
	Abs	4 exercises	1 set each to fatigue

Beginner: Second and Third Trimester Fitness

If you are healthy and do not develop any complications during your pregnancy, I would like to see you continue this workout regimen all the way through to delivery. Make sure you are using the Mommy Fabulous Pregnancy Modifications in this book and discontinuing any exercises you feel you can't perform correctly. If the two pound dumbbells are getting too heavy to maintain proper form, switch to one pound or use water bottles. You may want to add more time for stretching as pregnancy progresses.

Why does everyone keep talking about swimming during pregnancy?

Swimming is often recommended for many reasons. The first is that you are less likely to get hurt swimming. Second, activities done underwater tend to keep your heart rate and blood pressure lower than other forms of exercise. This makes swimming a good choice for someone with high blood pressure. Swimming can also be beneficial to those who develop swelling. When the body is underwater, the water pushes against the body creating what is called a hydrostatic force. If you have swelling, this force can help push the fluid that causes swelling back into the bloodstream. Getting in the water also feels good. As you get heavier, being underwater makes you feel lighter. Swimming can be both cardio and strength building; however it will not have the same benefits of weight bearing and core development that the Mommy Fabulous Program provides. Over all, swimming is a great activity because it works the whole body and I feel it is a great adjunct to the Mommy Fabulous exercises.

When I was pregnant, I would substitute a swimming workout when I was getting bored with my routine, or I would go swimming on days when I felt too tired to exercise. Swimming is exercise, but it never really felt like it… always a good thing!

Active Women
will fall into two categories: Intermediate or Advanced

- **Intermediate** would be those that currently exercise 3-5 times per week and probably think that some classes at the gym are too hard to participate in.
- **Advanced** are those that currently exercise 5-7 days a week and probably participate in a vigorous activity.

In the absence of obstetric or medical complications, most active women can continue to exercise at close to pre-pregnancy levels. Participation in sports such as volleyball and tennis, as well as aerobic exercise is generally safe during the first trimester. Weightlifting using appropriate weight is safe and effective. Some woman may be Advanced with regards to cardio but Intermediate in strength. You my have to customize your program based on both suggested regimens.

Running

Most runners can continue to run until late into pregnancy. Be aware that your performance will decline as pregnancy progresses. You should not attempt to maintain the speed, distance or time you were able to prior to pregnancy. Many runners continue to enjoy running but progressively shorten the length of time they do it.

Weight Training

A great deal of research shows weight bearing activities produce a number of benefits for women. The American College of Obstetrics and Gynecology lists weight training as a pregnancy exercise suggestion based on this research and because it has low to no impact on the joints. Relatively light weights and moderate repetitions will maintain flexibility and muscle tone while minimizing the risk of injury. Lifting of heavy weights should be avoided, except under professional supervision. For seasoned weightlifters, this is the perfect opportunity to modify your program or technique using the exercises in this book. Perform all sets and exercises for a specific muscle group one after another. Doing all your triceps sets and exercises consecutively before moving onto the next muscle or activity will ensure you get the maximum results. Between sets, rest for 30 seconds to two minutes. The more the muscle burns and fatigues the tighter and more beautiful it will be and the more calories will be burned. As pregnancy progresses, you will progressively lower the amount of weight you are lifting because maintaining proper form will become harder. During the third trimester, you may want to increase breaks towards two minutes to decrease the intensity of your workouts.

Sport Performance

As your pregnancy progresses, athletes should be aware that performance will decline. You should not attempt to maintain the speed, distance or time you were capable of prior to pregnancy. During the third trimester you should be especially cautious of sudden direction changes or quick changes in speed. Even if you are still capable, you can injure your joints due to the excessive momentum of your heavier body and the effects of joint laxity. Most athletes will voluntarily quit their sport six to eight weeks prior to delivery because they become ineffective workouts due to physical limitations. These sports include running, kickboxing and racquet sports among others. When you get to this point, don't be disappointed that you can not participate anymore. Be proud of yourself for sticking with it for so long and opt for another activity that will keep you in shape until you feel comfortable returning to your favorite sport. Practicing the Mommy Fabulous Program while pregnant will strengthen different elements of your fitness that may make you even more competitive after delivery.

Intermediate Fitness
Suggested First Trimester Regimen

1. Cardio: one hour, once to twice a week
   o Join a cardio aerobics class that meets weekly or biweekly.
     ▪ Great activities include step or spinning.
   o Or do a solo 45 minute to one hour cardio session once to twice per week.
     ▪ Great activities include jogging or speed walking, athletic conditioning, the rowing machine, the stair stepper or cycling.
2. Weightlifting using the Mommy Fabulous fitness techniques described in this book two to four times per week. Make use of the Easier or Advanced Modifications when appropriate.
   o You can substitute one weightlifting session for a weights class once per week, but be careful, these classes often do the reps too fast and with poor form. Let the instructor lead and then follow making your repetitions slow so the instructor does two for every one you do. Follow the form directions in this book. If you have never taken a weights class at a gym, I recommend avoiding them. You will get a safer, more effective pregnancy workout following Mommy Fabulous on your own.
3. Stretching: 30 minute session, once per week
   o Stretching should occur before and after every aerobic activity as well. Stretch between weightlifting sets instead of sitting. If you are active, you may not feel tight, but once you start stretching, you will find your limitations and imbalances. When you find one side of your body is more flexible, you need to correct this imbalance. This is why you need to dedicate a solid session to stretching at least once a week.
   o A prenatal yoga class can be helpful if it meets your interests.
4. Abdominals: 30 minute session, once per week
   o Ideally, abdominals should be challenged everyday. Keep abs engaged while doing aerobic activity. Mommy Fabulous exercises are all core focused. Adding three sets of ten, of any ab exercise at the end of each workout is a good way to stay on top of abs. At the very least, do a solid 30 minutes of abdominals every week.

Here is how it might look:

Sample Workout Regimen for the Intermediate Woman During the First Trimester

Day	Activity	Length of Time
Monday	Step Class	1hr
Tuesday	Weightlifting	45 minutes
	Abs	15 minutes
Wednesday	Stretch Session	20 minutes
	Abs	30 minutes
Thursday	Weightlifting	1 hr
Friday	Spin or Cycling Class **or**	1hr **or**
	Rowing Machine or Jog	30 minutes
Saturday	Weightlifting	45 minutes
Sunday	Stretch Session **or**	30 minute **or**
	Prenatal Yoga	1 hr

Sample Intermediate Weightlifting Breakdown

Day	Muscle Groups	Frequency	
Tuesday	Biceps	3 exercises	3 sets of 10 reps
	Butt & Thighs	4 exercises	3 sets of 10 reps
	Abs	4 exercises	2 sets of 10 reps
Wednesday	Abs	6 exercises	2 sets of 10 reps
Thursday	Chest	3 exercises	3 sets of 10 reps
	Shoulders	2 exercises	3 sets of 10 reps
	Hips	3 exercises	3 sets of 10 reps
Saturday	Triceps	3 exercises	3 sets of 10 reps
	Back	2 exercises	3 sets of 10 reps
	Calves	1 exercise	3 sets of 10 reps

Intermediate: Second and Third Trimester Fitness

- Weightlifting: As pregnancy progresses into the second trimester, you may need to start using the Mommy Fabulous Easier Modifications and decrease the weight to continue doing the exercises with good form. Discontinue exercises involving twisting or torso rotation; it taxes the lower back too much. Listen to your body, and you will know when you should start using the Pregnancy Modifications. You may want to spend more time doing the Mommy Fabulous exercises as they are low impact and shouldn't make you out of breath. As your cardio abilities decline as pregnancy progresses, you may want to increase Mommy Fabulous exercises from three days a week to four to six days a week doing fewer muscle groups per day, so the schedule might look more like the Advanced First Trimester Weightlifting Breakdown, except you would continue with the Intermediate Frequency column.
- Stretching: You will also want to dedicate more time to stretching as things begin to tighten up. Late in the second trimester I got a prenatal yoga video which I did occasionally when I felt really tight. By the end of the third trimester I was putting the DVD on at nine pm in a dimly lit room and doing the video once a week to meditate, stretch and prepare myself to sleep better. I did not substitute yoga for a workout; prenatal yoga was used as a stretch session.
- Cardio: It is usually the decreased ability to breathe (due to the baby crowding the diaphragm) that causes pregnant women to be discouraged by cardio activities. Take the intensity down, focus on taking deep breaths and try not to quit cardio altogether. Progressively make your cardio sessions shorter and more frequent.

Advanced Fitness
Suggested First Trimester Regimen

1. Cardio: One hour cardio once, preferably twice a week
   - Join a cardio aerobics class at least once a week, preferably twice if you aren't involved in a sport. Classes are better than solo cardio sessions because the activities will be balanced between upper and lower body and will be multidirectional as opposed to any cardio machine. If classes aren't your thing, reconsider during your pregnancy.

- Great activities include step, kickboxing, boot camp or dance.
  - Or participate in a sport once to twice a week
    - Great activities include tennis, rowing, non-contact martial arts or water polo because they balance upper and lower body involvement.
  - Or do a solo one hour cardio session once, preferably twice per week
    - Great activities include athletic conditioning drills such as jumping jacks, sprints, burpies, jump rope, etc.
2. Weightlifting using the Mommy Fabulous fitness techniques described in this book
   - Using proper technique, lift four to five times a week. Master the exercises and the Advanced Modifications in this book.
3. Stretching: 30 minute session, once per week
   - Stretching should occur before and after every aerobic activity. Stretch between weightlifting sets so you are not just sitting around. You need to dedicate a solid 30 minute session to stretching once a week. Even if you feel limber, this will reveal flexibility imbalances that need to be corrected. These will arise throughout your pregnancy.
4. Abdominals: 30 minute session, once per week
   - Abdominals should be challenged everyday. Accomplish this by keeping abs engaged while doing aerobic activity and practicing the core techniques of the Mommy Fabulous exercises. You may want to add three sets of ten of any ab exercise at the end of each workout or do one set of abs between weightlifting sets. Abdominals need a dedicated 30 minute session to really fatigue them.

Here is how it might look:

Sample Workout Regimen for the Advanced Woman During the First Trimester

Day	Activity	Length of Time
Monday	Kickboxing	1hr
Tuesday	Weightlifting Abs	45 minutes 15 minutes
Wednesday	Kickboxing Abs	1 hr 15 minutes
Thursday	Weightlifting	1 hr
Friday	Athletic Conditioning Drills Abs	30 minutes 30 minute
Saturday	Weightlifting	1 hr
Sunday	Weightlifting Stretch Session	30 minutes to 1 hr 30 minute

This schedule may sound intense, but it really wasn't hard. It only includes two hours and 30 minutes of sweat per week. The rest is working intelligently rather than hard. It is a time commitment, but you are worth it. Your baby is worth it. The health of you and your baby is worth the time working out. I was fortunate not to develop any pregnancy complications and was able to keep this routine until six weeks before my due date. I had a job, but I was able to take a nap during the day that helped keep my energy up.

Sample Advanced Weightlifting Breakdown

Day	Muscle Groups	Frequency	
Tuesday	Biceps	3 exercises	3 sets of 10 reps
	Hips	3 exercises	3 sets of 10 reps
	Abs	4 exercises	2 sets of 10 reps
Wednesday	Obliques	3 exercises	3 sets of 10 reps
Thursday	Triceps	3 exercises	3 sets of 10 reps
	Back	3 exercises	3 sets of 10 reps
Friday	Abs	6 exercises	2 sets of 10 reps
Saturday	Chest	3 exercises	3 sets of 10 reps
	Butt & Thighs	4 exercises	3 sets of 10 reps
Sunday	Shoulders	3 exercises	3 sets of 10 reps
	Butt	1 exercise	3 sets of 10 reps
	Calves	1 exercise	3 sets of 10 reps

Advanced: Second and Third Trimester Fitness

- Weightlifting: As pregnancy progresses into the second trimester, you may need to start using the Mommy Fabulous Easier Modifications and decrease the weight to continue doing the exercises with good form. Discontinue any exercises involving twisting or torso rotation. Listen to your body, and you will know when you should start using the Pregnancy Modifications. When my cardio abilities declined as pregnancy progressed, I increased Mommy Fabulous exercises from four days to six to seven days a week doing fewer muscle groups per day. See chart on the following page.

- Stretching: You will want to dedicate more time to stretching as things begin to tense up. Late in the second trimester I got a prenatal yoga video that I did occasionally when I felt really tight. By the end of the third trimester, I was putting the DVD on at nine pm in a dimly lit room and doing the video once a week to meditate, stretch and prepare myself to sleep better. I did not substitute yoga for a workout; prenatal yoga was used as a stretch session.

- Cardio: At about week 34, six weeks prior to my due date, I could not keep up with the kickboxing even going at a much slower pace, avoiding some moves and modifying others. I then substituted the stair stepper three to four times a week for 30 minutes. You could also switch from a vigorous cardio activity to a cycling or spin class and go at your own pace. But I gotta tell you, six weeks on a stair stepper gives you a gorgeous ass and thighs. On days when I was too tired to do more, I walked on the treadmill or swam.

Headed to the gym
Week 39

Sample Workout Regimen for the Advanced Woman During the Third Trimester

Day	Activity	Length of Time
Monday	Biceps	30 minutes
	Abs	10 minutes
	Cardio (stair stepper)	30 minutes
Tuesday	Triceps	20 minutes
	Hips	20 minutes
	Stretch Session (before bed)	20 minutes
Wednesday	Shoulders	30 minutes
	Abs	10 minutes
	Cardio (stair stepper)	30 minutes
Thursday	Chest	35 minutes
	Calves	5 minutes
	Stretch Session (before bed)	20 minutes
Friday	Back	30 minutes
	Butt & Thighs	30 minutes
Saturday	Abs	10 minutes
	Cardio (stair stepper)	30 minutes
Sunday	Swimming	30 minutes
	Stretch Session (prenatal yoga)	1 hr

Mental Preparedness

Staying fit is not easy. Being pregnant is not easy. Being a woman is not easy. Combine all three and you have a hell of a lot of work ahead of you. Mental preparedness is going to become very important in your life. You are mentally gearing up for labor, to be a mother to this new child, a new life, a new title. You need to be mentally prepared for this program as well. You must believe that you are worth this time and effort. You must commit to your health. You must believe that fitness will benefit your baby. I bet you would do anything to give your baby the best chances for health… including working out. I often hear people say, "Yeah, I know exercise is important, but I'm tired." There is a difference between knowing something is true and *believing* something is so important that it is a choice-motivating factor. There were many days I was in the gym because I loved my daughter, not because it was what I felt like doing.

Chapter 14

The Exercises

Do NOT just follow the pictures. Read the instructions. There is a lot of subtle positioning involved in doing these exercises with good form that can be overlooked when just imitating a picture. Small adjustments, of any kind, will increase or decrease efficiency and the safety associated with the movement. Don't be intimidated by the nit-picky descriptions of form, I want to protect your back and knees. The descriptions are meant to be helpful and answer questions my pregnant clients ask.

Each exercise is first introduced for a woman of Intermediate fitness in her first trimester. Modifications are then given to make the exercises **Easier** for the fitness Beginner, and **Advanced** modifications show you how to make the exercises more challenging. Once you have mastered an exercise, it may only take a small adjustment to make the exercise more challenging. There are modifications specific for the second and third trimesters called **Pregnancy Modification**. Trimester safety ratings are listed in the upper right of each exercise description as well as in the Exercise Index. An **X** represents each trimester. Three **XXX**s indicate that the exercise can be safely performed, with modifications, during all three trimesters. For exercises that require traditional gym equipment, I also included **Variations** that show you how to perform the same exercise without gym equipment. All these exercises can be done in a gym or at home with a minimal amount of equipment.

Equipment Needed if Not Using a Gym

If you don't belong to a gym or want or workout at home occasionally, I recommend that you buy four to five pieces of equipment. Any brand of equipment will work fine.

1. BODY BALL		Cost ~ $12 from discount store, $24-50 retail
		The ball diameter should be equivalent to your knee height.
2. RESISTANCE BAND		Cost ~ $5.50 from discount store, $12-15 retail
		preferably with jump rope handles
3. DUMBBELLS		Cost $6-15 per set retail
	Beginners	2 pound set needed for all fitness levels
	Intermediate	2 pound set and 5 pound set
	Advanced	2 pound set, 8 pound set and 15 pound set
4. BAR		Cost $25 - $60 retail
	Beginners	9 pound bar like those made by SPRI
	Intermediate	9 to 15 pound bar
	Advanced	9 to 25 pound bar

Must Have Item

The body ball is the single most important piece of exercise equipment you should have in your home during your childbearing years. Even if you workout in a gym, having a body ball in the house provides more opportunity for stability training to develop core strength. Sit on the ball while watching TV. Practice lifting one foot off the floor. During my third trimester I sat on the ball instead of a chair at dinner and when on the computer. It was infinitely more comfortable because it keeps you from slouching which causes your back to get sore. After delivery I would sit on the ball and work my abs while rocking Talia; she loved it! They are not expensive and you will get a lot of use out of it. Choose a body ball with a diameter equivalent to your knee height. A 65 cm ball is probably the best for someone who is 5 foot 8 inches tall. A 55 cm might suit a person who is 5 foot 4 inches tall. If you are 5 foot 2 inches tall, a 45 cm ball would probably be best. Pick one up at a discount store, online, used sport shop or borrow one.

Every person's waistline expands at a different rate, and each person develops different pregnancy related issues. This is only a guide, not a judge of your abilities. Some women will start the program as a beginner and with practice and dedication may move onto the **Advanced** modifications during the second trimester then during the third trimester she will do the **Pregnancy Modifications**. Some will start the program doing the **Advanced** modifications and move to the **Easier** and then **Pregnancy Modifications** as pregnancy progresses. You may find that you can handle some of the **Advanced** modifications in some exercises and only the **Easier** modifications in others, highlighting muscle imbalances. Maybe you will be intermediate through the whole pregnancy. I don't care where you are or where you end up on the spectrum. If you do the program consistently, regardless of the level, you will recover from this pregnancy looking better than ever. If at any time, you feel like your posture is straining to keep good form, simply move onto the next modification even if you have not progressed into the next trimester. For exercise to be efficient and as safe as possible, proper form is critical.

All of these exercises are designed to challenge your core. In order to get the most out of the program you must master the Pelvic Tilt first (page 113). Doing these same exercises throughout your pregnancy will continue to be challenging because you will be gaining additional weight, and changing physically. You are chasing a moving target! Begin this program immediately! If you wait too long to start these exercises, even the **Easier** modifications may become too difficult for you. A pregnant woman who has been balancing on one foot for 30 weeks straight will find these exercises challenging, fun and safe. A woman 30 weeks pregnant who has been running for years but has never stood on one foot may feel unstable because her core, hips and foot muscles are weak. Being physically fit does not mean you will be conditioned for this type of exercise, so start this program now and perform the exercises often.

Finally, do NOT choose from the Exercise Index. This is not a menu. This is not a program where you only do the exercises that are easy for you. Likewise, just because you like the way your calves look, doesn't mean they do not need to be exercised. The Mommy Fabulous workout is a balanced program designed so that you don't end up with some strong muscles and some weak ones. As discussed previously, muscle imbalances lead to aches, pains and injuries. If an exercise causes discomfort because you can't seem to position yourself properly or painful due to a previous injury, then skip it by all means. You just want to be aware that you are not spot training a certain muscle group and that the goal here is to explore exercises outside your usual program. As you progress in your pregnancy you will need to decrease the amount of weight and intensity of your workouts. This is the opposite of how a person would train if they were not pregnant. You should feel good about this, because, remember, you are *carrying* more resistance.

Core Exercise Index

Abdominal tone must be maintained throughout the entire pregnancy for an easy, speedy recovery to a tiny waist and a flat stomach. Unlike other muscle groups, abs can be exercised everyday.

Trimester Safety Recommendation*

Core Exercises	First Trimester	Second Trimester modify as needed	Third Trimester modify as needed	Page
Self Check Diastasis Recti	X	X	X	102
Correction of Diastasis Recti	X	X	X	102
Pelvic Tilt	X	X	sitting or standing position	103
Kegel	X	X	X	104
Plank	X	X		105
Modified Mountain Climber	X	X		105
Lumber Jack Ball Rotation	X	discontinue		106
Wood Chopper	X	discontinue		107
London Bridges	X	discontinue		108
Lying Leg Circles	X	limit time lying on floor		109
Crunch	X	limit time lying on floor	modify on ball or Bosu	110
Ball Crunch	X	X	X	111
Crunch with Knee Cross	X	limit time lying on floor		112
High Knees	X	X	X	113
Front Kicks	X	X	X	114
Serenity Abs	X	X	X	115
Oblique Lateral Knee Raises	X	X	X	116
Bicycle	X	limit time lying on floor		117
Side Plank	X	X		118
Accordion Side Crunches	X	X	X	119

* If any exercise becomes too difficult to maintain proper form, move on to the Easier or Pregnancy Modification.
* If any exercise causes pain, discontinue immediately.
*Modifications of abdominal exercises are necessary for women who develop diastasis recti.

Exercise Index

Trimester Safety Recommendation*

Exercise	Muscle Group	First Trimester	Second Trimester modify as needed	Third Trimester modify as needed	Page
Standing Straight Arm Lat Pulldown	Back	X	X	X	120
Lat Pulldown		X	X	decrease weight	121
Upper Back Extension		X	modify to standing	modify to standing	122
Lower Back Extension		X	may need modification		123
Standing Back Kick	Butt	X	X	X	124
Standing Rear Leg Lifts		X	X	X	125
Gluteal Pendulum		X	reduce range of motion		126
Reverse Lunge	Butt & Thighs	X	X	reduce range of motion	127
Stationary Lunge		X	X	reduce range of motion	128
Stationary Side Lunge		X	X	reduce range of motion	129
Adductor Machine		X	X	X	130
Booty Bridge		X	X	modify on ball	131
Squat		X	X	reduce range of motion	132
Sumo Squat		X	X	X	133
Adductor High Knees		X	X	X	134
Lying Adductor Leg Lifts		X	X	X	135
Side Chamber	Hips	X	X	X	136
Side Kicks		X	X	X	137
Sea-Saw Kicks		X	X	X	138
Abductor Machine		X	X	X	139
Fire Hydrant Back Kicks		X	X	X	140
Bench Press	Chest	X	X	X	141
Dumbbell Flye		X	X	modify on ball	142
Push Ups		X	may need modification	modify or discontinue	143
Burpy		X	may need modification		144
Lateral Shoulder Raises	Shoulders	X	X	decrease weight	145
Standing Up and Over		X	X	modify to no weight	146
Shoulder Flye		X			147
Seated Overhead Dumbbell Press		X	X	decrease weight	148
Seated Triceps Extension	Triceps	X	X	decrease weight	149
Triceps Dips		X	X	modify	150
Skull Crusher		X	X	decrease weight	151
Cable Rope Triceps Extension		X	X	decrease weight	152
Standing Dumbbell Bicep Curl	Biceps	X	X	decrease weight	153
Hammer Curls		X	X	X	154
Concentration Curl		X	X	decrease weight	155
Twenty-Ones		X	X	decrease weight	156

* If any exercise becomes too difficult to maintain proper form, move on to the Easier or Pregnancy Modification.
* If any exercise causes pain, discontinue immediately.

Stability Challenge Exercises

Stability exercises are important so that you reduce your chance of losing your balance as pregnancy progresses. They improve posture, body awareness and core strength while increasing joint stability. They also help to prevent feet from spreading or developing flat feet by keeping the muscles in the feet toned. Always perform these exercises slowly and with the safety of a sturdy chair nearby.

Trimester Safety Recommendation*

Exercise	Muscle Group	First Trimester	Second Trimester modify as needed	Third Trimester modify as needed	Page
Calf Raises	Calves	X	X	X	157
One Leg Calf Raise		X	X	X	157
Standing Back Kick		X	X	X	124
Standing Rear Leg Lifts	Butt	X	X	X	125
Gluteal Pendulum		X	reduce range of motion		126
Reverse Lunge		X	X	reduce range of motion	127
Booty Bridge	Butt	X	X	modify on ball	131
Adductor High Knees	&	X	X	X	134
Side Chamber	Thighs	X	X	X	136
Side Kicks		X	X	X	137
Bench Press on a body ball		X	X	X	141
Dumbbell Flye on a body ball	Chest	X	X	modify on ball	142
Push Ups		X	may need modification	modify or discontinue	143
Triceps Dips	Triceps	X	X	modify	150
Plank		X	X		105
Crunch on a body ball		X	X	X	111
High Knees		X	X	X	113
Front Kicks	Core	X	X	X	114
Serenity Abs		X	X	X	115
Oblique Lateral Knee Raises		X	X	X	116
Side Plank		X	X		118
Accordion Side Crunches		X	X	X	119

*These stability challenge exercises are safe for pregnant women, but not all balance exercises are. These exercises should be performed slowly and cautiously. Use your judgment and don't push yourself if you don't feel secure. Always have a sturdy chair or wall to support yourself with or grab onto if you lose your balance.

* If any exercise becomes too difficult to maintain proper form, move on to the Easier or Pregnancy Modification.

* If any exercise causes pain, discontinue immediately.

Floor Work
The "I'm Tired" Workout

Perform these exercises while lying on the floor or sitting cross legged in front of the couch with your back supported by the couch. When you are tired, do these exercises slowly. Take long breaks between sets. Do them while watching TV instead of just vegging. You will feel more limber and energized if you do something rather than nothing.

Trimester Safety Recommendation*

Exercise	Muscle Group	First Trimester	Second Trimester modify as needed	Third Trimester modify as needed	Page
Booty Bridge	Butt	X	X	modify on ball	131
Rear Leg Lifts (pregnancy modification)		X	X	modify to lying	125
Lying Adductor Leg Lifts	Inner Thighs	X	X	X	135
Adductor Machine (ball modification)		X	X	X	130
Abductor Machine (variations)	Hips	X	X	X	139
Sea-Saw Kicks		X	X	X	138
Fire Hydrant Back Kicks		X	X	X	140
Up and Over (sit cross legged)	Shoulders	X	X	eliminate weight	146
Lateral Shoulder Raises (sitting)		X	X	eliminate weight	145
Pelvic Tilt	Core	X	limit time lying on floor	sitting or standing	113
Kegel		X	X	X	114
Serenity Abs		X	X	X	115
Crunch		X	limit time lying on floor		110
Crunch with Knee Cross		X	limit time lying on floor		112
Oblique Lateral Knee Raises (leaning on chair variation)		X	X	X	116 117

* If any exercise causes pain, discontinue immediately.

Core Exercises

You should check yourself for diastasis recti before you begin these core exercises and you should self-check once a week throughout your pregnancy.

Self-Check for Diastasis Recti   **XXX**

Starting Position: Lie on your back, with your knees bent and feet on the floor. Place your fingers over your belly button.

Execution: Lift your head off the floor. Measure the width of the separation between the abdominal muscles with your fingertips. If you can place more than two fingers in the muscle gap, you have diastasis recti and you need to modify the core exercises. Learning to do a pelvic tilt correctly is imperative to prevent and improve this condition. The Pelvic Tilt is described on the next page.

Correction of Diastasis Recti

Starting Position: Lie on your back, with your knees bent and feet on the floor.

Execution: Exhale as you rock your pelvis back and flatten the lower back into the ground (pelvic tilt) then tuck your chin, and slowly raise your head off the ground while pushing the ab muscles toward the midline with your hands. Do not try to lift shoulders off the floor. Inhale as you slowly lower your head and relax.

Variation: Fold sheet lengthwise under your low back. Cross sheet over your abdomen, holding opposite ends in each hand. As you tuck your chin and raise your head, pull outward on the ends of the sheet to cinch your waist. As you lower your head and relax, release the grip on the sheet.

Pregnancy Modification: Avoid exercises that require lying backward over a large exercise ball (none in this book), avoid all exercises that cause your abdominal wall to bulge outward upon exertion (draw abs inward), avoid exercises were you twist like racquet sports. Women who develop diastasis recti and are 12 weeks or more into the pregnancy should avoid aggressive abdominal exercise as it may make the condition worse. Discuss this with your doctor.

Pelvic Tilt

This is the single most important technique that will give you a fabulous stomach for life. It is sometimes referred to as *drawing the navel to the spine.*

Standing Variation

Starting Position

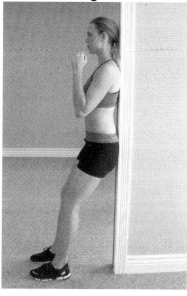

Execution

Starting Position: Lie on your back, with your knees bent and feet on the floor. There should be a small natural arch in your lower back. Arms and hands should be relaxed, lying on the ground.

Execution: Exhale as you press the lower back into the floor by drawing your abs to your spine. This will cause your pelvis to tilt backward. Hold for five seconds. Inhale as you slowly relax the abdominal muscles.

Tips: You can tilt the pelvis by contracting your butt muscles, but this is totally pointless. Your butt checks should be completely relaxed and the abdominal muscles from your belly button to your pubic bone should be contracting. Lie relaxed and think about pulling your pubic bone towards your chin.

Variations:
Once you get the hang of how to do a pelvic tilt while lying on the ground, practice while sitting in a chair, while standing and then on a body ball.

Pregnancy Modification: After week 20, you should not lie on your back for extended time. Practice the variations often.

Easier: Not sure if you are doing it right? Place a ruler under the small of your back at rest, so that you can feel your back pressing into it during the execution.

Advanced: Draw your shoulder blades together underneath you. This causes the lower back to arch upwards more. Then use the lower abdominal muscles to flatten your back to the floor. Hold for 10 seconds. Master holding a pelvic tilt while taking several breaths without relaxing the contraction.

Kegels

Starting Position: You can do Kegel exercises any time, any place and in any position. Try sitting on the floor leaning backwards on your hands. Keep the spine straight. Knees should be bent with feet flat on the floor spread wide.

Execution: Inhale as you contract the pelvic floor (see Tips) visualizing an elevator rising up floors. Exhale as you release. The butt, hamstrings and inner thighs should remain relaxed. Contract the pelvic floor muscles and hold for 10 seconds, then relax them for 10 seconds. Breathe continuously through the contraction. Repeat 5 to 10 times. These muscles fatigue quickly. Perform three times per day.

Tips: Learn how to control the muscle by stopping the flow of urine, but do not continue to practice doing this as it may lead to a urinary tract infection. Another way to locate the muscle is to practice squeezing the penis during sex. You will feel the muscle tighten around the penis so you will know you are doing the exercise correctly.

No pregnancy exercise regimen would be complete without discussing the Kegel. The muscles that make up the pelvic floor support the organs from sagging onto the bladder and vagina. These muscles have a heavy burden with the baby pressing on them. Many pregnant women experience urinary incontinence when the pelvic floor muscles are weak. This doesn't usually just go away after birth as labor also stretches the pelvic floor. The Kegel exercise strengthens the pelvic floor muscles. If you already have urinary incontinence, practicing Kegels will help. You should follow the routine suggested above because if you overwork the pelvic floor it could worsen the problem. You don't want to over- Kegel. In addition to preventing urinary incontinence, strong pelvic floor muscles also enhance sex. These muscles are the same muscles that squeeze or grip the penis. Now I know most of you don't want to be thinking about exercise while you are having sex, but I could never really figure out if I was doing the dang exercise. You know you are doing it during sex, so do a few reps during sex to get the hang of it. When the pelvic floor muscles are strong the sexual sensation is better. Major plus!!!

Plank

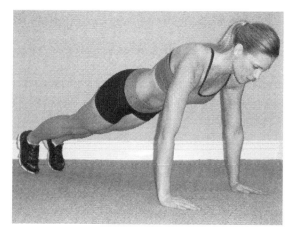

Starting Position: Get into a push up position on the floor with your hands directly under the shoulders and the feet shoulder width apart. Focus on a spot on the floor about 18 inches away.

Execution: Draw the naval to the spine to get your body straight from head to heels. Hold the plank as long as your abs can support your back from sagging downward.

Tips: Do not lift the butt upward; use the abs to keep the body straight. Don't drop the head, it makes a plank harder to hold, but not in a good way.

Variations:

Pregnancy Modification: As the weight of the baby begins to strain the lower back, increase the incline you perform the exercise at. Place hands on a bench at the gym. At home, place hands on stairs, a windowsill or on a counter. Discontinue exercise when the weight of the baby strains the lower back.

Easier: Perform a plank on your hands and knees. Or rest your elbows and forearms on the ground. You can start in a full plank and drop the knees to the ground when your back begins to strain to work on extending plank hold time.

Advanced: Place the feet together. Work up to holding a plank for 1 minute.

Modified Mountain Climber

Starting Position: Begin in the plank position.

Execution: Three part move: Using the abdominal muscles, draw the right knee toward the right elbow as you exhale. Inhale as you tap the right toe back at the starting position. Exhale as you draw the right knee toward the left elbow. Inhale as you tap the right toe back at the starting position. Exhale as you rotate the right leg outward at the hip (dog at a fire hydrant) and draw the right knee toward the right elbow. Inhale as you tap the right toe back to the starting position to complete one rep. Switch legs.

Tips: The Modified Mountain Climber takes the jumping and jarring out of a mountain climber, making it safer on joints and for pregnancy. Think of it as a high knee, a cross high knee and an oblique lateral high knee.

Variations:

Pregnancy Modification: As the weight of the baby begins to strain the lower back, increase the incline you perform the exercise at. Place hands on a step, then on a bench, then on a counter, then on a wall. When the size of your belly interferes with the exercise, stop doing the cross knee. Slow it way down. Discontinue exercise when you can not perform the exercise without straining your back.

Easier: Perform this exercise with arms on a bench or a Smith Machine bar set at waist level or on a counter. The greater the incline, the easier it is.

Advanced: Performing this exercise on the ground is hardest. Maintain a flat back and work on speed. Perform 10, and then switch legs.

Lumber Jack Ball Rotation

Starting Position

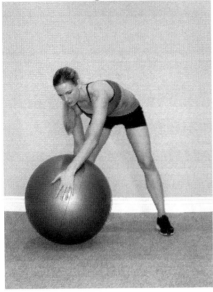

Execution

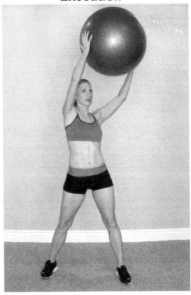

Starting Position: Stand with your feet wider than shoulder width apart with the right foot six inches behind parallel. Place a body ball in front of your right foot. (Ball diameter should be knee height.) Draw your naval to the spine and bend over to the right at the waist. With extended arms, place the left hand in front of the ball and your right hand behind it.

Execution: Four part move, done as a single fluid motion: 1) Exhale as you contract the left oblique pulling the torso up to standing. 2) When you get to a normal standing position, rotate the arms so that the right hand is now on top of the ball and the left hand in underneath it. 3) Continue the path of the ball up and over your left shoulder. Use your right oblique to stop the momentum of the ball. 4) Draw your abs forcefully toward the spine to pull the torso back through the rotation to starting; you should feel a good ab crunch here. Perform 5 then switch sides.

Tips: Imagine you are a lumberjack and the ball is a tree stump. Pick up the piece of wood and throw it over your shoulder into the truck behind you. Do not twist your hips too much, try to keep abdominal control.

Variations:

The motion can be done with any light weight ball like a soccer ball, but if you are using a small ball, you should tap it to your knee, not the ground.

Pregnancy Modification: Discontinue during the second trimester when the back becomes less mobile. Twisting will result in pulled back muscles.

Easier: Don't bend over as far. You don't have to tap the ball to the ground. In fact, you can still work the abs without bending over at all. Just do the arm motion while keeping the abs tight.

Advanced: The more you mentally focus on your abs, the more you can make the rest of your body NOT help them. This will make the ball feel heavier. Perform 10 reps on the right, followed by 10 on the left and you should get a good cardio workout. Don't use a weighted medicine ball because it changes the exercise from core isolation to a back and arm workout.

Wood Chopper

Starting Position

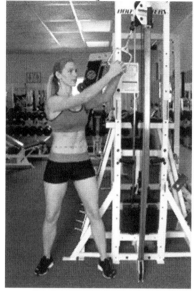

Execution

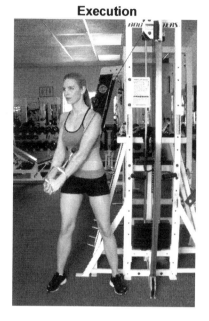

Starting Position: Get into a wide stance with feet parallel to the cable. Twisting at the waist, place your body weight on the foot closest to the cable. Hold one cable handle in both hands, with the far hand on top. Arms and wrists should stay straight through the move, and the hands should be centered in front of your chest. Draw your navel to your spine.

Execution: Exhale as you rotate your upper body pulling the cable diagonally downward toward the opposite knee, while shifting your body weight to the other foot. Hold an abdominal contraction for a beat. Inhale as your abs resist the cable tension and slowly rotate back to the starting position. Do not let the weight plates touch down.

Tips: The hands should be centered in front of your chest the whole time, the arms do not move, only the torso moves at the waist. This exercise is more about what is *not* moving. From the starting position, imagine the contracted core is like a corset that does not wanting to move, but the upper body rotation is forcing it. From the execution position, think about the core not wanting to return to the starting position. This exercise is most effective when done at a snail pace.

Variations:
This exercise can be performed by using a resistance band connected to something taller than you.

Pregnancy Modification: Discontinue during the second trimester when the back becomes less mobile. Twisting will result in pulled back muscles.

Advanced: Try to keep your hip bones stationary and squared. Try to isolate the abdominals when you are twisting.

London Bridges

Starting Position

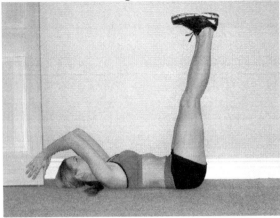

Execution

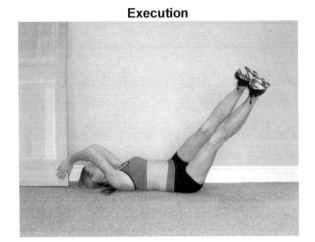

Starting Position: Lay flat on the ground in front of a couch leg or a sturdy table leg or any heavy stationary object. Draw your shoulder blades down and together underneath you. Grab the stationary object with both hands; elbows should be pointing toward the ceiling. Draw your navel to your spine and flatten your lower back to the floor. Bring your legs up so they are together, straight and perpendicular to the floor (as much as possible). Pull toes downward so feet are parallel to the ceiling. This exercise is ideally performed on a weight bench. Grasp the bench under your head.

Execution: Keeping the feet flat and together, inhale as you allow your abs to stretch by letting the legs drop to the right in a slow and controlled manner. Only drop the legs down as far as you can while keeping them straight and keeping your back pressed flat into the floor. Exhale as you slowly pull the legs back to starting by forcefully drawing the abs to the spine. Alternate directions.

Tips: Be sure that there is no momentum. The lower back should never rise off the floor. If you can't get your legs straight, work on stretching your hamstrings. If they are tight now, they will negatively affect your abilities later and may cause back pain in your third trimester.

Variations: At the gym, perform these lying on a flat bench while holding onto the bench near your head.

Pregnancy Modification: Discontinue exercise by week 20. Do not perform if you develop diastasis recti.

Easier: Practice holding the starting position for 10 seconds forcefully pushing your back into the floor. This is hard work too! Drop the legs only a few inches. Do not drop the legs if it hurts your lower back.

Advanced: Work up to performing 20 continuous reps, 10 on each side, alternating direction.

Starting Position

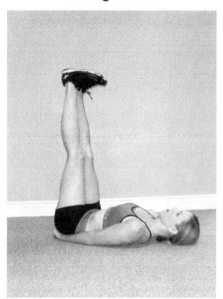

Starting Position: Lie on your back with your knees bent, feet flat on the ground. Pull your shoulder blades down and together underneath you. With your palms facing down, cup your hands and place them under your butt checks and raise your legs into the air. Keep the feet together and flexed so they are parallel with the ceiling. Draw the navel to the spine pressing the back flat into the floor.   Your cupped hands will keep your pelvis tilted through the move.

Execution: Inhale as you slowly lower the legs down as far as you can without your back lifting off the floor. At this point exhale as you spread the feet and legs outward and forcefully drawing the abs toward the spine, pull the legs back in an arc to the starting position. The legs should make individual circles while keeping the feet flat.

Execution

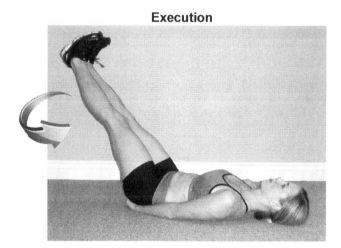

Execution

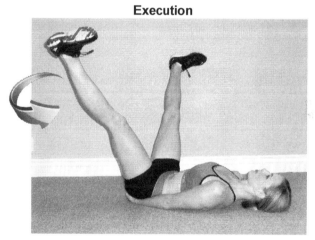

Variations:

Pregnancy Modification: Follow the Easier modification. After week 20, do a set and then rest on your side. Discontinue exercise when the weight of baby strains lower back.

Easier: Size doesn't matter…at least in this case. Only drop the legs a few inches and make the circles small. It's more important to keep the back flat on the floor than the size of the circles.

Advanced: The wider you spread the feet, (i.e. the larger the leg circles), the harder it will be, plus you will work the inner thigh muscles. If you can raise your head and shoulder blades off the ground without using your neck muscles, do it. It takes a lot of core strength and muscle control to keep the neck relaxed in this position, but it is actually easier to keep the lower back on the ground allowing a greater range of motion.

Crunch

Starting Position

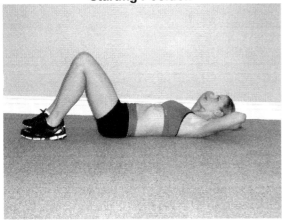

Execution

Starting Position: Lie on your back with your knees bent and feet flat on the floor at shoulder width apart. Draw your shoulder blades down and place your hands under your neck and cradle your head off the ground as dead weight. Your elbows should be directly outward from the body. Draw your navel to your spine, flattening your back on the floor. Abs should be tense.

Execution: Exhale as you forcefully pull the belly button downward into the floor, lifting the shoulder blades off the floor about 1-3 inches. You should aim your chin at the spot where the wall meets the ceiling. Inhale as you slowly set the shoulder blades back on the ground. Do not let the lower back lift off the ground, or set the head down. Repeat.

Tips: Look at the spot where the wall meets the ceiling so that you are not tempted to curl your head toward your chest. Placing hands under the neck rather than behind the head will also help to keep your spine straight. Do not use your neck muscles, your head should be dead weight in your hands. You are lifting your upper body toward the ceiling, not curling your head toward your knees. Your butt and thighs should be relaxed.

Variations:

Pregnancy Modification: Limit time on your back after the 20th week. Perform a set and then rest on your side. Discontinue the crunch on the ground when you are no longer comfortable and move onto the Ball Crunch or perform crunches on a Bosu.

Easier: Practice holding the starting position. Practice taking several breaths without letting your back pop off the floor.

Advanced: Lift the shoulder blades 3 inches off the ground without rounding the spine.

Ball Crunch

Starting Position

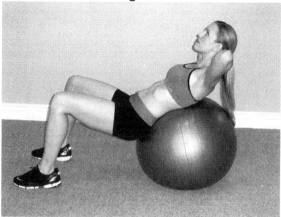

Execution

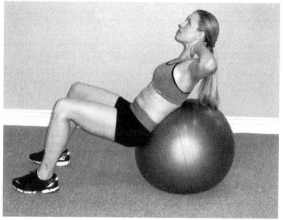

Starting Position: Sit on a body ball in good posture. Walk you feet forward, rolling out until the bottom of your shoulder blades touch the ball. Then do a pelvic tilt. Relax the neck and keep the spine properly aligned. Place hands behind the neck and cradle the head with the elbows directly outward from the body. Your abs should be working to keep your body from tipping backwards.

Execution: Exhale as you forcefully draw the navel to the spine. (This will **cause** your upper body to rise forward a few inches.) Keep the spine straight. Aim your chin to the spot where the wall meets the ceiling. Inhale as you slowly resist gravity as you return to starting. Repeat.

Tips: The abs never get to rest. The range of motion is small. Look at the spot where the wall meets the ceiling so that you are not tempted to curl your head toward your chest. Do not use your neck muscles. You are lifting your upper body toward the ceiling, not curling your head toward your knees.

Variations:
This crunch can also be performed on a Bosu by sitting on the edge.

Pregnancy Modification: None needed. Spread feet wider if needed.

Easier: Placing your feet further apart gives you more stability. Practice doing these with your toes pushed up to a wall until you are comfortable stabilizing yourself on a body ball. Keep the range of motion to a few inches. The higher you sit on the ball the more stability you will have.

Advanced: A larger range of motion does not make a crunch more effective. If you have a strong core, you should probably be able to crunch the abs about one foot from the top to the bottom of the move while keeping a straight back and a pelvic tilt. To increase the challenge, squeeze a 2 lb. medicine ball or a big stuffed animal between your knees.

Crunch with Knee Cross

Starting Position

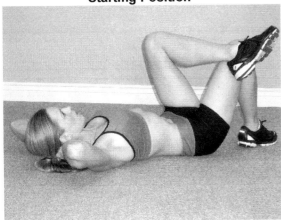

Execution

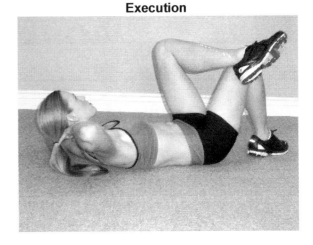

Starting Position: Lie on the ground with knees bent and feet flat on the floor at shoulder width apart. Cross the legs by placing the left ankle on the right thigh just below the right knee. Draw your shoulder blades down and place your hands under your neck and cradle your head off the ground as dead weight. Your elbows should be directly outward from the body. Draw your navel to your spine, flattening your back to the floor.

Execution: Exhale as you forcefully pull the belly button downward into the floor lifting the right shoulder blade off the floor 1-3 inches. You should aim your right shoulder at the spot where the wall meets the ceiling. Inhale as you slowly set the shoulder blade back on the ground but do not let the lower back lift off the ground. Perform 10 reps then switch legs and sides.

Tips: The elbow should remain directly out from the shoulder. The shoulder joint should not move; you are not touching your elbow to your knee; you are lifting your shoulder blade toward the ceiling. Keep your eyes on the spot where the ceiling meets the wall so that you don't curl the neck forward.

Variations:

Pregnancy Modification: After week 20, do a set and then rest on your side. Discontinue exercise when the size of the belly interferes with the exercise or do the Advanced modification.

Easier: Do fewer reps.

Advanced: Rather than discontinue this great move during advanced pregnancy, (if you have good balance) move this exercise to a body ball. Keep both feet on the ground spread wide, instead of crossing them. Perform 10 basic crunches, then 10 crunches to the right, followed by 10 crunches to the left to complete one set with no break. Keep the crunches small, you must maintain a straight back and a pelvic tilt.

High Knees

Execution

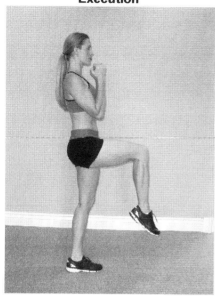

Starting Position: Stand in good posture with weight on the left foot and the knee slightly bent. Keep the right knee bent as you balance. Pull your shoulder blades down and back. Your hands should be held in front of your chest in two fists held next to your chin as a boxer, or placed together as if your were praying. Do a pelvic tilt which will rock your torso backwards a bit. Pull naval toward the spine.

Execution: Exhale as you use your abs to raise your right thigh. The lower leg and foot should be relaxed. Inhale as you lower the right leg. Only lower as far as you can keep your abs engaged and your back straight.

Tips: If you feel like you are hunching forward, put your hands behind your neck and keep your elbows pointed outward from your body.

Variations:

Pregnancy Modification: None needed. As your belly gets larger, the knee may not be able to get as high, but this is a great exercise to perform all the way through pregnancy.

Easier: Place two sturdy chairs on each side of you to grab for balance.

Advanced: Perform 10 high knees on one leg. Without breaking, get into the execution position as your new starting position and pulse the leg up 2 inches as you exhale and return to waist height as you inhale. Perform 10 pulses and then switch legs.

Front Kicks

Execution Step 1 & 3

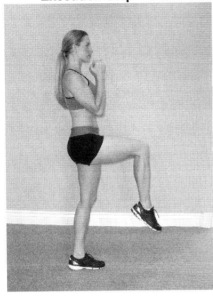

Execution Step 2

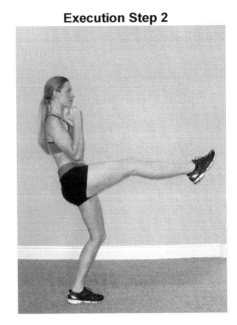

Starting Position: Stand in good posture with weight on the right foot and the left foot a half step in front with the knee bent and the left toe touching the ground. Pull your shoulder blades down and back. Your hands should be held in front of your chest in two fists held next to your chin as a boxer, or placed together as if you were praying. This stating position is the same starting position pictured in the Reverse Lunge.

Execution: 4 part move: 1) Inhale as you step onto the left foot transferring all your body weight and performing a right High Knee. 2) Exhale as you quickly snap the lower right leg forward fully extending the knee joint with a pointed toe. 3) Quickly snap the lower right leg back to the high knee position. 4) Release the abs and quickly step down onto the right foot. Return to starting by transferring all the weight to the right foot and picking up the left heel. Perform 10 reps and then switch legs.

Tips: The hip bones should stay level and pointed forward. Stretch the butt and hamstrings to get greater range of motion. Front kicks will also work the quads, so stretch the front of your thighs too. A side or back kick can be done slowly, but a front kick should be a faster, smooth motion. Focus on using your abs to lift the leg, rather than the leg muscles.

Variations:

Pregnancy Modification: None needed. As your belly gets larger, the kick will not be as high, but this is a great exercise to perform all the way through pregnancy. You will also get slower.

Easier: It does not matter how high your high knee or kick is. It only matters that you are using you abs to lift the leg. Practice doing the high knee to gain strength.

Advanced: These can be performed as 20 alternating leg front kicks. Or you can do 10 right front kicks without transferring weight from the left leg. These can be a great cardio drill.

Starting Position & Execution

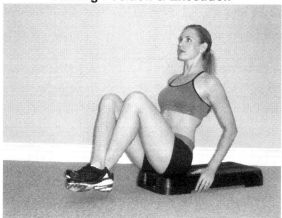

Starting Position: Sit on the edge of a bench in good posture. Perform a pelvic tilt, which will rock your torso backward a bit. Your abs should be working to keep you from tipping over backward. Pull your shoulder blades down and back. Your spine should be straight from head to tailbone. Inhale.

Execution: Exhale as you draw both knees up towards your chest. The inner edge of your shoes should be touching, or you can cross your ankles, but the knees should be comfortably spread. Hold as long as you can, practicing deep even breathing, focus, concentration and pulling the abdomen inward. Can you find serenity?

Tips: Focus on relaxing the whole body and letting the abs do the work. Make your abs hug your baby as hard as they can.

Variations:

Pregnancy Modification: None needed. Spread the knees wider to accommodate your baby belly. When or if your abs can't support your back, move to the Easier modification.

Easier: Perform this exercise while sitting on the floor. Only your tailbone and heels should be on the floor. The wider apart and further away your feet are from the body, the easier it will be. To make it even easier, prop yourself up with pillows until your back is straight and try to NOT use the pillow support as much as you can.

Advanced: Sit on top of a Bosu to perform this exercise. For the ultimate challenge, put your hands behind your neck in crunch position or hold your hands to the outside of your body, palms facing the ceiling in a mediation pose.

Oblique Lateral Knee Raises

Starting Position

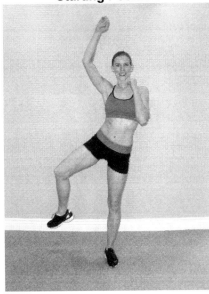

Execution

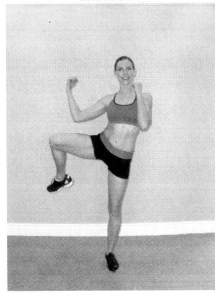

Starting Position: Stand in good posture with weight on the left foot and the knee slightly bent. Bend the right knee and rotate the right leg outward at the hip, so the knee is pointed to the right. The right foot should be relaxed. Pull your shoulder blades down and back. Pull naval toward the spine. This is the starting position.

Execution: Exhale as you contract the right oblique (side of the waist) using it to raise the right leg into a lateral high knee.

Tips: The hips and shoulders should stay squared and parallel with the floor.

Variations:

Pregnancy Modification: None needed. Hold onto a tall backed chair placed on your left side for stability. Do the sitting variation on days when you are tired.

Easier: Don't do the arm motion, it makes balancing harder. Hold onto a tall backed chair placed on your left side for stability. Tap the right foot on the ground between reps and don't raise it as high.

Advanced: Perform 10 high knees with each leg. Then, with no break, raise the right knee to waist height and pulse it up 2 inches as you exhale and return to waist height as you inhale. Perform 10 pulses then switch legs.

Sitting Variation:

Sit on the floor with a chair or couch seat under your left armpit. Sit on your left hip with your left leg lying on the floor with the knee bent. Rotate the right leg so the knee and shoe laces are pointed toward the ceiling by drawing the knee toward the right shoulder. Your right oblique should be squeezed. Execute by extending the right leg and pushing with the right heel. Keep the foot flexed. The leg should rotate so the knee and shoe laces are facing forward. The oblique will have to work to keep the leg up.

Tips: The hips and shoulders should stay squared and pointing forward. Make these easier by tapping the right heel on the ground. Try not to lean on the chair.

Oblique Lateral Knee Raises

Starting Position   **Execution**

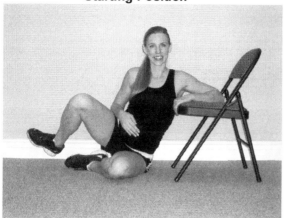   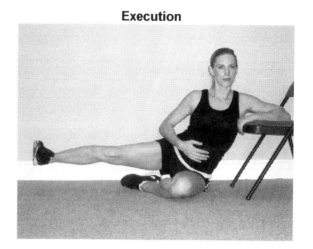

Bicycle

Starting Position: From a crunch starting position, bring the feet off the floor by pulling the knees to the chest.

Execution: Exhale as you extend your left leg out straight, while simultaneously lifting the left shoulder off the ground and aiming your left elbow over your right knee. Inhale as you release the abs allowing the shoulder blade to return to the floor. Exhale as you quickly switch the leg positions repeating the move by bringing the right elbow over the left knee. The low back should stay pressed into the ground.

> **Tips:** Most people aim their elbow at the knee, if you aim it up and over the knee, you will get better core results. Keep the elbows open wide. Going too fast is less effective; practice control.

Variations:

Pregnancy Modification: After week 20, do a set and then rest on your side. Discontinue exercise when it becomes uncomfortable.

Easier: Extend the legs toward the ceiling instead of straight out. Aim your foot for the spot where the wall meets the ceiling.

Advanced: Instead of discontinuing bicycles, you can sit on the end of a bench if your abs are strong enough to keep your back straight. Place your hands softly on the bench behind your butt and draw your legs up balancing on your tailbone (Serenity Abs position). Then extend the right leg as you exhale. Inhale as you draw the leg back up. Repeat with the left. It is okay to go slowly and spread the knees to accommodate a baby belly.

Side Plank

Advanced Execution

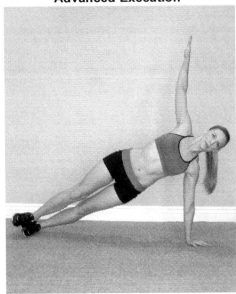

Starting Position: Lie on your left side, resting on your left elbow with your forearm resting on the ground in front of you. Your feet, hips and shoulders should be stacked on top of each other. Draw your navel to your spine.

Execution: Exhale as you contract the left oblique (the left side of the waist) lifting your hips off the floor until your body is straight from head to feet. Hold and then inhale as you slowly return to starting.

> **Tips:** It is easy to let the hips and shoulders roll forward or backward; keep these joints stacked.

Variations:

Pregnancy Modification: Follow **Easier**. Discontinue when the weight of the baby strains your lower back or the exercise feels uncomfortable.

Easier: Perform the side plank at an incline by placing the left hand on a bench to make it easier. Or get into the starting position by lying on the floor and resting on your elbow and forearm instead of your hand. Bend your left knee 90 degrees, so that the knees are together, but the lower left leg is lying on the ground behind you. Keep your right leg straight and rise into a side plank keeping the lower left leg on the ground to help lift some of the weight by pressing it into the floor.

Advanced: Perform the side plank on your hand instead of the elbow. Work up to holding the plank for a minute. From the side plank position, dip your left hip downward, stretching the oblique (left side of the waist) and then contracting it to pull the body back up into a plank. Do not set the hips back on the ground. Perform 10 reps, and then switch sides.

Accordion Side Crunches

Starting Position

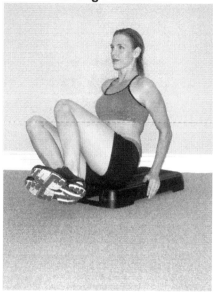

Starting Position: Sit on the edge of a bench on the left butt check. Both butt bones should be to the right. Place your hands behind you on the bench for stability and to help you keep a straight back. Draw the naval to the spine. Inhale as you draw the knees up towards the left shoulder and breast. Keep the feet flexed with the toes pulled up.

Execution: Exhale as you extend the legs, pushing through the heels. Only extend the legs as far as you can keep the abs contracted. Inhale as draw the knees back to the starting position.

> **Tips:** Your torso will rock forwards and back between the starting position and execution; this is fine as long as you keep your back straight.

Execution

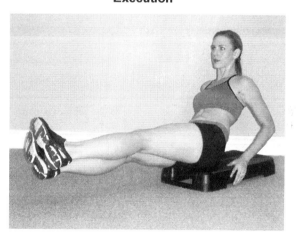

Variations:
These can be performed on the ground, on a bench, on a chair or on a Bosu.

Pregnancy Modification: None needed. Do this on a bench or Bosu and spread the knees wider to accommodate a growing belly. Make the range of motion small to protect the back, the legs do not need to fully extend.

Easier: Perform these on the ground. Tap the lower heel down when the legs are extended and when the legs are drawn close to the body. To develop strength, hold the starting as long as you can. Perform pulses with a small range of motion to gain strength.

Advanced: Perform these while sitting on top of a Bosu. Place your hands behind your neck for the ultimate balance challenge.

Standing Straight Arm Lat Pulldown   XXX

Starting Position

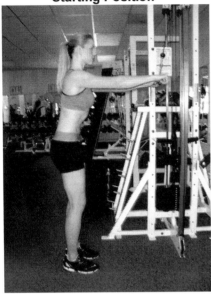

Execution

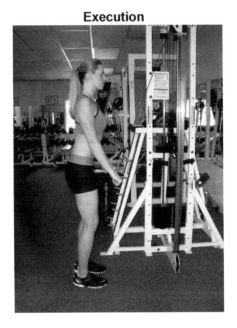

Starting Position: Stand in front of a cable machine with a straight bar attachment. Feet should be shoulder width apart, hips and knees should be slightly bent. Torso should be bent slightly forward at the waist. Bring the abs to the spine. Elbows and wrists should be straight with hands spaced on the bar a little wider than shoulder width apart. In the starting position, the bar and hands should be about shoulder height.

Execution: From the starting position, exhale as you use your upper back muscles to pull the bar downward. Keep all joints, except the shoulder, in the same position through the whole move. Bring the bar down until it is a few inches from the thigh. Inhale as you slowly resist the cable and return to starting. You should feel the upper back muscles stretching as you return to starting, but do not allow the weight plates to touch.

Tips: This exercise is for the muscles that cover the shoulder blades. Keeping your elbows pointed outward, instead of down, keeps tension on the lat muscles. Keep your head and waist in the same position. Do not watch the bar, and do not bend forward at the waist as you lower the bar. If you do not keep your abs pulled toward your spine, your back will over-arch causing stress in the lower back.

Variations:
This exercise can also be done by a using a resistance band attached to something taller than you. Or a closet dowel, securely attached to resistance bands can be substituted for a bar and cable machine.

Pregnancy Modification: You will have to decrease the weight as pregnancy progresses so the lower back is not strained. Discontinue when your abs become too weak to stabilize your lower back.

Lat Pulldown

Starting Position

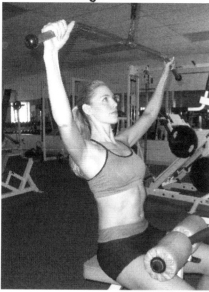

Execution

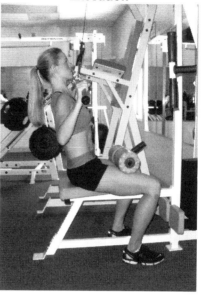

Starting Position: Sit at the Lat Pulldown machine with knees at 90 degrees and ankles under the knees. Grasp the bar just outside the bend keeping the wrists straight. Elbows should be slightly bent and pointed outward from the body. Do a pelvic tilt, leaning the torso back slightly until your abs are contracted to keep you from falling backward. The spine should be straight from head to tailbone. This is the *resting* position. Now use the upper back muscles to pull the shoulder blades down. This is the starting position.

Execution: From the starting position, pull the bar downward by using your upper back muscles to rotate the shoulder blades around and down until the shoulder blades are pinched together. The elbows will lead the arms in an outward and downward arc until the elbows are slightly behind the waist and the hands are in front of the shoulders. You should be sitting upright enough that the bar will come very close to your nose as you pull it down past your face to your chest. While the bar should not touch your chest, it should come down to an inch or two below your collar bone.

Tips: Use your abs to stabilize your body, not your lower back. There is a tendency to contract the lower back, and it should be relaxed. Don't cheat! You should not be using any arm muscles to perform this exercise. The farther the bar is from your nose, the more you will be using your arm muscles instead of your back. The **Lat**, as in *Lati*simus Dorsi, is an upper back muscle. In the execution position, you should be squeezing an imaginary finger between your shoulder blades. Keep the head aligned with the spine. Do not watch the bar.

Variations:

A closet dowel, securely attached to resistance bands can be substituted for a bar and cable machine. Sit on a body ball and hook the resistance band on something overhead. You can also perform the same motion using resistance bands without the closet dowel.

Easier: Use lower weight or perform this exercise with resistance bands hooked to something overhead.

Pregnancy Modification: You will have to decrease the weight as pregnancy progresses so the lower back is not strained. Discontinue when your abs and upper back muscles become too weak to stabilize your lower back.

Upper Back Extension

Starting Position

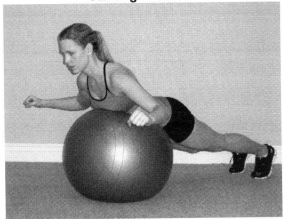

Execution

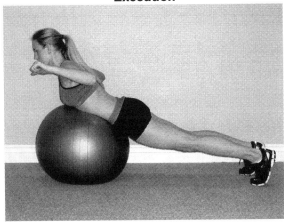

Starting Position: Place your rib cage on a body ball or Bosu so that your nipples are touching the ball, but are not smashed on it. Head should be aligned with the spine, so you should be looking at the floor. Arms should be relaxed outwards so that wrists and elbows are just a little lower than the height of the shoulders. Elbows should be bent and hands relaxed.

Execution: Exhale as you use the muscles of the upper back to pull the shoulder blades together. This should cause your breasts to lift off the ball or Bosu and your arms to rise until the elbows and wrists are just about shoulder height. Inhale as you slowly return to starting without letting the upper back muscles go completely limp.

Tips: Your lower back should remain relaxed through the move; it is not lifting the upper body. Bending the knees, rather than keeping them straight, can help to keep your lower back from getting involved. The vertebrae in your back and neck should not change position much. You are moving your shoulder blades not your spine. Have someone place their finger between your shoulder blades and try to squeeze it. Keep your neck and shoulder muscles relaxed.

Variations:

Pregnancy Modification: Discontinue using a ball or Bosu when you no longer feel comfortable lying on your stomach. Perform the exercise in the standing position. Take a large stride backwards with one foot (execution of Reverse Lunge) and place the majority of your weight into the front foot. Keeping good spinal alignment, perform the arm motion described above.

Easier: Use a Bosu, or place your heels against a wall to give you more stability on the ball. Placing your feet wider apart will also give you more stability. The lower you let your arms fall between reps, the easier the exercise will be...it will also be less effective. Challenge yourself.

Advanced: Hold the shoulder blade squeeze for 3 seconds before slowly lowering. Perform 3 sets of 10 reps.

Lower Back Extension

Starting Position

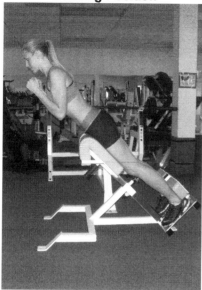

Execution

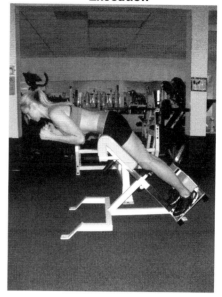

Starting Position: Place your feet on the platform with toes pointed straight ahead, in line with the knees. The hip bones should be just above the thigh pad. Knees should be slightly bent and the body should be straight from head to heels. Your hands should be in front of your chest in two fists held next to your chin as a boxer. Because you are holding your body straight, your lower back should already be contracted.

Execution: Inhale as your lower back muscles resist gravity and slowly lower your upper body. Lower your upper body until your lower back muscles are staining to hold your torso; if you drop further the lower back muscles will become lax and uncontracted. Exhale as the lower back muscles contract, slowly pulling the torso upwards until it is completely straight from head to heels. Do not hyperextend the back by pulling up too far. This move should be smooth and slow through the whole range of motion, do not use momentum to elevate the upper body.

Tips: Do not hold a weight. Your upper body already weighs a lot and people who use a weight tend to move too quickly through the move because the upper body plus a weight is too heavy and they end up not doing that much work overall. If your breasts are heavy, criss cross your arms over your chest using your arms to support the breasts. Be sure to keep your butt and thighs relaxed, they shouldn't help.

Variations:

Pregnancy Modification: As the lower back becomes more taxed and less mobile as pregnancy progresses, use a smaller range of motion. Lower your upper body only a few inches and slowly return to starting. Criss cross your arms across your chest to support the breasts if they feel heavy. You will need to discontinue this exercise when the weight of baby strains the lower back. The starting position may be all the work you need.

Advanced: Do not hold a weight; for an added challenge, place your hands behind your head with the thumbs pointed down the neck and elbows pointed outwards from the body. If these seem easy after 3 sets of 10, you are using momentum and gravity rather than the lower back.

Bosu Variation: During the first trimester, the reverse movement can be performed by all fitness levels, while lying on the floor or on a Bosu. Lay on a Bosu with your hips on top. Place bent elbows and forearms on the ground for support, and keep the head aligned with the spine. Tighten the lower back to lift the legs up off the floor. To avoid using the butt muscles, keep knees slightly bent with feet in a neutral, relaxed position. The further you spread the legs apart as they rise, the less the glutes will be used and the more the lower back will be isolated.

Standing Back Kick   XXX

Starting Position	Step 2 & 4	Step 3

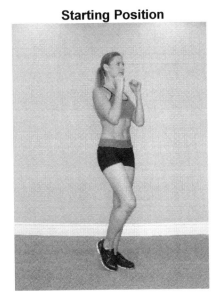 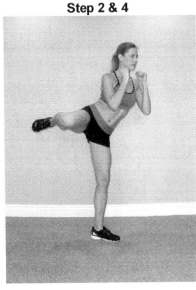 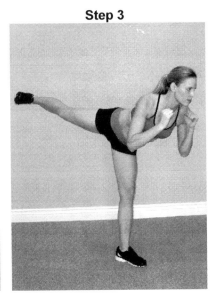

Starting Position: Stand upright in good posture with weight on the left foot with the knee slightly bent. Pull your shoulder blades down and back. Your hands should be held in front of your chest in two fists held next to your chin as a boxer, or placed together as if you were praying. Arms should not change position during this exercise. Pull naval toward the spine.

Execution: 5 part move: 1) Starting position. 2) Inhale as you bend forward at the waist and use the right hip muscle to lift the right leg out to the side while simultaneously bending the knee and pulling the toes forward. Do not raise the knee any higher than you can raise your foot. 3) Leading with the right heel, exhale as you forcefully extend the leg backwards as if pushing someone. When the leg is fully extended the right glute should be squeezing hard. 4) Pull the leg back in using the hip muscle by bending the knee. 5) Return to starting by taping the right foot back to the ground with total control (no gravity) and standing up straight. Switch legs.

Tips: You should not be using your lower back for this move. If you feel the low back muscles, lean forward more, contract the abs tighter and focus on the hip and glute muscles. The hips and shoulders should be squared forward, do not allow the body to roll open to the right. This move requires stretching. The stiffer your leg muscles are, the harder it will be to balance.

Variations:

Pregnancy Modification: Place a tall backed chair in front of you and place your hands just above the chair to grab when you need support. This is a great exercise to practice concentration and balance. It is very important that you keep the spine aligned while pregnant, twisting at the torso places too much stress on the back. There is no twisting in this kick. During the third trimester the belly can have a weight of its own. I kept the right fist at my chin, and the left arm wrapped under my belly (pictured in Side Chamber).

Easier: Break this move down. Hold onto a chair and perform very slowly to build strength. Don't try to raise your leg as high as the picture. Do not raise the knee any higher than you can raise your foot. Practice step 2 until your hip is strong enough to lift your leg without using your back or obliques. Practice step 3 holding onto a chair until your glutes are strong enough that your back doesn't get involved. Then practice putting the steps together.

Advanced: Perform 10 reps on each leg slowly with total balance and control. Then perform 10 reps on each leg working on speed, balance and control for a cardio workout. If you have completely mastered form and control and have great balance, you can add a set of 20 where you alternate legs for each kick. Discontinue alternating or slow down considerably during the third trimester.

Standing Rear Leg Lifts

Starting Position

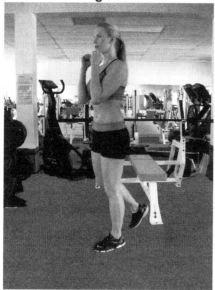

Execution

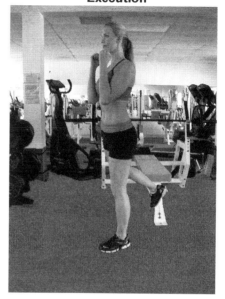

Starting Position: Stand upright in good posture with weight on the left foot with the knee slightly bent. The right leg should be behind you with the foot in a neutral, relaxed position. Pull your shoulder blades down and back. Your hands should be held in front of your chest in two fists held next to your chin as a boxer, or placed together as if your were praying. Pull naval toward the spine. Use the right glute (butt check) to raise the right leg an inch off the ground.

Execution: Exhale as you tighten the right glute raising the right leg. The leg will rise back and outward, diagonally from the body. Both hip bones should be squared with the shoulders and pointed forward. Do not let go of your pelvic tilt. Inhale and slowly control the glute allowing the right toe to lightly tap the ground.

Tips: The hardest part is keeping the hips from *opening up* to the right. A solid pelvic tilt prevents this. The right toe should be able to raise no more than 6-10 inches off the ground. If you can get yours higher, then you are arching your back or leaning forward. It is so easy to do these quickly and let gravity lower the leg. Control your own butt!

Variations:

Pregnancy Modification: None needed. Have something to grab onto for safety. It may be nice when you feel tired to do these lying on the floor. You don't get the core benefits of weight bearing and balancing, but at least you can work the butt. Fold up your left arm and lay your head on your left forearm on the ground. As your belly gets larger you may want to lay along side a pillow and place your belly on top of it for support. You may need to roll forwards a bit to isolate the glute, just be sure to keep the hips and shoulders aligned; don't twist at the waist. Perform the leg lifts backward and upward making sure your lower back remains relaxed.

Easier: Place a tall backed chair in front of you and place your hands just above the chair to grab when you need support. This is a great exercise to practice concentration and balance.

Advanced: Perform 10 reps. Then rotate your leg inward at the hip so that the knees are closer together and the right toes point downward. The heel leads this leg lift. The range of motion will be smaller for these lifts, but you will feel a solid glute squeeze.

Advanced Execution

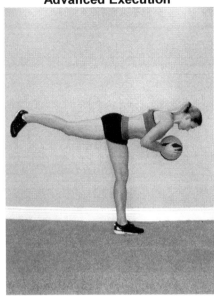

Starting Position: Stand in good posture with weight on the left foot with the knees slightly bent. Pull your shoulder blades down and back. Your hands should be held in front of your chest in two fists held next to your chin as a boxer, or placed together as if your were praying. Pull naval toward the spine. The spinal alignment including shoulders, hips and neck should stay constant through the move.

Execution: Imagine your whole body is a straight board from head to the right ankle. Inhale as you slowly allow the left butt muscles to stretch as your upper body lowers by leaning forward at the left hip and the right leg elevates. Stop tipping at the point (just before) where you can't keep your body straight. Both hip bones should be squared with the shoulders and pointed directly downward. You should feel a maximal stretch in the muscle were your left butt check meets your thigh. Now exhale as you contract it to bring the whole body back to the starting position. Switch legs.

Tips: This exercise is hard and takes tremendous concentration as well as good balance to perform correctly. The hardest part is keeping the hips from *opening up* to the right. Notice that the knee cap is pointed down toward the ground. Many people use their lower back to return to starting. You must use your mind to relax the back and use only your left glute. Balance is in the core, keep your abs contracted. This move requires hamstring stretching. The stiffer your leg muscles are, the harder it will be to balance and the smaller range of motion you will be capable of.

Variations:

Pregnancy Modification: Perform this exercise with your hands on two sturdy chairs placed on either side of you. Decrease the range of motion as the belly interferes with the move. Even if you only get the leg off the ground twelve inches while keeping the body straight, the glutes will get an amazing workout. You will need to discontinue the exercise when it strains the back (due to the increased weight of the torso or the weakening of the stretched abs) or when you can not keep proper form due to the size of your belly, whichever comes first.

Easier: You must be comfortable standing on one foot to practice this move. If your balance is good, but not great, perform this exercise with your hands on two sturdy chairs placed on either side of you. Reduce the range of motion. Even if you only get the leg off the ground twelve inches while keeping the body straight, the glutes will get an amazing workout. Perform 5 correctly on each leg. Even if you can not do these well, working on your balance is beneficial for your muscles and for your safety during daily life.

Advanced: During the first trimester, if you have amazing balance, you can hold a medicine ball or weight (no more than 3 pounds) against your chest with both hands and perform the exercise. Perform 3 sets of 10 reps on each leg. If you feel you can do more weight, you are doing the exercise incorrectly. Discontinue using the weight once you are *showing* as your torso will have gained weight to make up for it.

Reverse Lunge   XXX

Starting Position

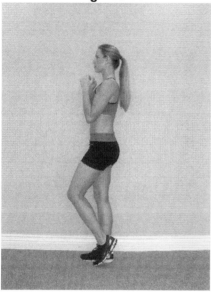

Execution

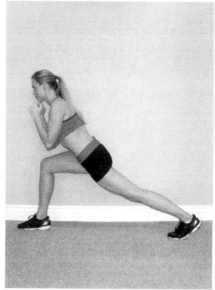

Starting Position: Stand in good posture with weight on the right foot with the knees slightly bent. Pull your shoulder blades down and back. Your hands should be held in front of your chest in two fists held next to your chin as a boxer, or placed together as if your were praying. Pull naval toward the spine.

Execution: Inhale as you step backwards with the left leg, bending the right knee until the right thigh is parallel with the ground. Only the ball of the left foot should touch the floor. Again, activate the core as you exhale and push the body weight through the heel of the right foot as you rise back into the starting position.

Tips: Head, neck and spine should align. Do not add weights. Holding a barbell behind your neck will place too much downward force on your spine. Holding dumbbells in the hands will cause your shoulders to roll forward and cause your back to compensate for the less than perfect posture. Your body weight should remain in your right heel through the whole move. Forward lunges place a lot of stress on the knees, I never advise them.

Variations:

Pregnancy Modification: If you are having trouble keeping good posture as the body moves, place a closet dowel behind your head, and hold each side with your hands. This keeps the upper body aligned properly. Reduce range of motion as your belly expands. Discontinue when the size of your belly interferes with the exercise.

Easier: Do not lunge as deep. Go down as far as you can keeping the body straight from head to heel until you are strong enough to get your thigh parallel to the floor.

Advanced: Get into the starting position on a step. Perform the reverse lunge by stepping backwards off the step. When returning to standing, don't push off with the left leg, force the right leg to do all the work.

Stationary Lunge

Starting Position

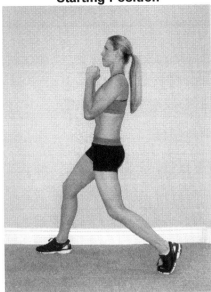

Execution

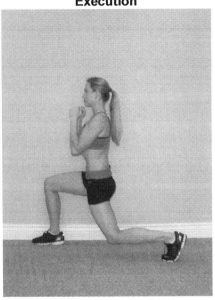

Starting Position: Step your left leg backwards larger than one stride length and much wider than shoulder width apart. Pull your shoulder blades down and back. Your hands should be held in front of your chest in two fists held next to your chin as a boxer, or placed together as if your were praying. Perform a pelvic tilt; you will need to bend your left knee and bring your left heel off the ground. Your left knee should be under your hip and line up with your head.

Execution: Inhale as you bend the right knee, and lower the body directly down until your right thigh is parallel with the floor. Exhale as you press the majority of your weight into the ball of your left foot. You will feel most of the work in the front of your left thigh. Perform 10 and switch legs.

Tips: Do not lean forward; you should be vertical from head to knee. The right knee should not travel forward over your toes. If it does, step the left leg back farther and wider. The pelvic tilt protects your back and isolates the muscle in the front of the thigh, the quad.

Variations:

Pregnancy Modification: Reduce the range of motion as your belly expands. Discontinue when the size of your belly interferes with the exercise.

Easier: Shoot for 5 reps on each leg done correctly. Place chair backs on each side of you so you can use your arms to assist you on the way up. You will gain more strength doing the full range of motion with arm assistance over doing small ranges of motion.

Advanced: Play with where you distribute your body weight, 60% on the ball of the left foot, then 75%. The more weight you put in the back foot, the harder it will be.

Stationary Side Lunge

Starting Position

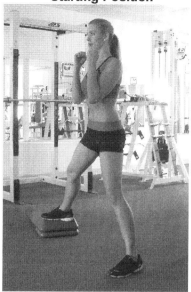

Execution

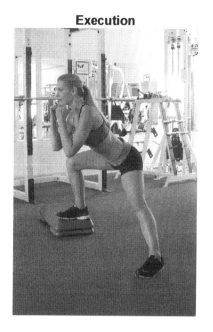

Starting Position: Place your right foot on the edge of a step. Stand with feet parallel and wider than shoulder width apart. Legs should be straight with a slight bend in the knee and all your weight should be in your heels. Pull your shoulder blades down and back. Your hands should be held in front of your chest in two fists held next to your chin as a boxer, or placed together as if you were praying.

Execution: Inhale as you bend the right knee sitting backward into the lunge until the right thigh is parallel with the floor transferring your body weight to the right leg. The left leg should remain straight but the knee should not be locked. The torso will lean forward in this lunge. Head, neck and spine should align with natural curve in the lower back. As you exhale, push the body weight through the right heel, straightening the right leg and rise back into the starting position. Perform 10 reps and then switch legs.

Tips: The shoulders and hips should stay aligned and pointing forward...no twisting. Keep the arms close to the body; extending the arms forward will cause you to fold yourself in half at the waist. As the knee bends, it should not move forward over the toes, the body should go backwards and the knee should stay in the same place.

Variations:

Pregnancy Modification: Reduce range of motion as belly expands. Discontinue when the size of your belly interferes with the exercise.

Easier: Place the arch of the right foot on the edge of a step that is no more than 1 foot tall. Perform lunge to the right. This helps makes the range of motion smaller.

Advanced: Place the foot on the side of a Bosu instead of a step.

Adductor Machine

Starting Position: Sit down in the machine upright or leaning slightly forward. Use the lever to adjust the foot pedals out as far as your thighs will spread apart comfortably. Lock the lever and then sit back into the seat. You will need to tilt your pelvis back in order to press your lower back into the seat. If there is a head rest, use it.

Execution: Exhale and slowly squeeze the inner thighs together until the knees just touch. They should not come crashing together; you must control the machine, not the other way around. Inhale as you slowly resist the tension as the machine pulls your knees back apart. Do not let the weight touch down.

Tips: The inner thigh muscle should never be resting during the whole set. It should go from being stretched to contracting, but not resting.

Variations:
This exercise can be done using a body ball instead of a machine. Sit on the edge of a bench or chair and place the body ball between the knees and squeeze. Make sure your feet are spread wider than your knees. Slowly release but only so far as there is still inner thigh muscle tension. These can also be performed on the ground in the Kegel starting position.

Pregnancy Modification: None needed.

Easier: Use less weight and a smaller range of motion. Do not let the inner thigh muscle rest during the set by letting the weights touch together or releasing tension on the body ball.

Advanced: Keep adding more weight for each set. This machine is safe through pregnancy as long as you press your lower back into the seat. Perform this program with the body ball variation: Perform 10 squeezes slowly as described, on the last one hold the squeeze for 7 seconds, squeezing harder for 3 seconds more then do an additional 10 at regular pace. Ten second break. Next perform 10 squeezes, then perform 20 pulse squeezes were the movement is fast and small, perform 5 squeezes at normal pace.

Booty Bridge

Execution

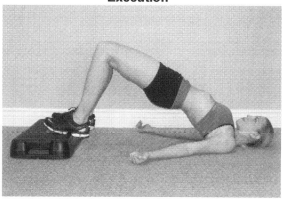

Starting Position: Lie on your back with the arches of your feet on the edge of a step. (You want to be close enough to the step so that when you are in the bridge position, your knees are at a 90 degree angle.) Pull your shoulder blades together underneath you and use your glutes to lift your hips off the ground a few inches.

Execution: Exhale as you press your arches into the step, lifting your hips as high as you can. Ideally you should get your body straight from knees to shoulders. Squeeze the butt hard at the top and slowly lower until your hips are a few inches off the ground. Do not set the hips down on the ground...no resting!

Tips: Do not press your hands into the floor, arms should be relaxed. As your butt gets fatigued, your knees will drift apart, don't let them! You may want to do this next to a mirror so you can see if you are bridging high enough. As the glutes get tired, the butt will lower and the bridge won't be as straight. This is **not** one of those exercises you should quit when form declines. This is an exercise a pregnant person can and should power through.

Variations:

Execution with Pregnancy Modification

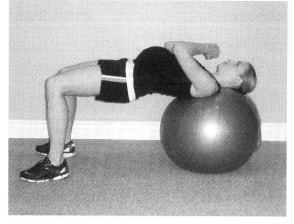

Pregnancy Modification: Perform on a body ball. Sit on the ball and then walk your feet outwards until your head and shoulders are resting on the ball. Bridge upwards until your body is parallel with the floor. Your knees should be at a 90 degree angle, so that your ankles are directly under the knees with feet flat on the ground. The wider you set your feet apart the more stability you will have on the ball. My back looks arched in this picture, by it is an illusion because my butt and belly are bigger.

Easier: Set the hips down on the ground between each rep. It gives the glutes time to rest. It is better to do this and perform a solid bridge than to keep the hips elevated and perform a lazy set.

Advanced: Perform 10 bridges as described, on the last one hold the bridge up for 10 seconds squeezing hard. Next perform 5 bridges, then perform 10 pulse bridges were the movement is fast and small, finally perform 5 normal bridges. There is no rest in this set.

Advanced Challenge: Place only your heels on the top of the Bosu. Perform 10 booty bridges. For the second set, lift the right leg and point it straight up toward the ceiling. With the left heel on the Bosu, perform 10 single leg booty bridges. Then switch legs. You may not be able to bridge as high on a single leg bridge. Be sure to keep your hips parallel to the floor. Do not perform a single leg booty bridge while on a body ball; it is not safe.

Squat

Execution

Easier & Pregnancy Modification

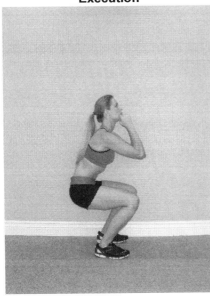

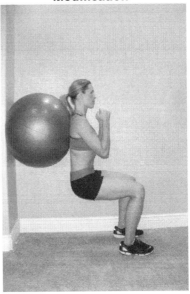

Starting Position: Stand with your feet just outside shoulder width apart and angled outward about 20 degrees. All your weight should be in your heels. Pull your shoulder blades down and back. Your hands should be held in front of your chest in two fists held next to your chin as a boxer, or placed together as if your were praying.

Execution: As the knees bend, the body should go backwards while trying to stay upright. The knee should not move forward past the toes. When the upper thighs are parallel with the floor, tuck the pelvis forward by doing a pelvic tilt. Then exhale, contract the core and begin to ascend back to the starting position by pushing all your weight through your heels. Hands and arms should remain motionless.

Tips: Most people extend the arms and chest forward, folding themselves in half at the waist- so no work is done. Cross your arms in front of you with your elbows at shoulder height like a geinie. Balance a closet dowel across them and perform the squat without letting the dowel roll off your arms. This will help to keep you upright and not leaning forward. As you stand up out of the squat, look at the ceiling and lift your chest upward. The pelvic tilt protects your back from arching and isolates the thigh muscles.

Variations:

Pregnancy Modification: None needed. Do wall-ball squats. Place a body ball against a wall in the small of your back, and perform the squat as described. As you squat down, the ball will roll up your back. It is easier because you can press some of your body weight into the wall. You must perform a pelvic tilt at the bottom of the execution or your lower back will arch (your butt will follow the ball). As your belly gets bigger, reduce the range of motion. Try not to spread the legs to accommodate the stomach.

Easier: Practice getting up and sitting down on a seat using proper squat form. Practice doing a smaller range of motion rather than the full range incorrectly. As your legs get stronger you will be able to do the full range. Or do wall-ball squats.

Advanced: Do not add weights, this will tax your back and usually makes people lean forward to offset the weight. Master the technique (especially the pelvic tilt) and this will continue to get harder as you gain weight. You know you have mastered a squat when you can do one facing a wall with your toes about two inches from the wall.

Sumo Squat

Starting Position

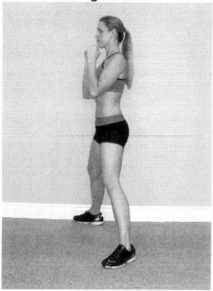

Execution

Starting Position: Place your feet out wide enough so that when you are in the execution position and your thighs are parallel to the floor, your knees are over your ankles. Angle the feet outward. Your hands should be held in front of your chest in two fists held next to your chin as a boxer, or placed together as if your were praying. Pull naval toward the spine.

Execution: Inhale as you bend the knees and push the hips backward, lowering your body until your thighs are parallel with the floor. With your legs in this position, you should be able to do this without leaning forward much, if at all. Exhale as you squeeze the inner thighs together to raise the body. Your weight should be in your heels.

Tips: Keeping abs tight prevents the back from arching. This squat should be felt in the inner thighs. To activate the inner thighs, imagine you are trying to pull your knees together but your feet are stuck in cement.

Variations:

Pregnancy Modification: None needed.

Easier: Do a smaller range of motion. Don't go down as far.

Advanced: As you rise out of the squat to the starting position, squeeze the lower butt checks hard. It is like doing a pelvic tilt with the butt instead of the abs. This is an awesome exercise and will get harder as pregnancy progresses, but will always be safe.

Advanced Challenge: After you master the sumo squat, perform the sumo squat on the ball of the right foot and keep the left flat on the ground. After 10 reps, switch the elevated heel. After 10 reps, do 10 sumo squats on the balls of both feet. This technique is for the quads rather than the inner thigh. Do all variations.

Adductor High Knees

Starting Position

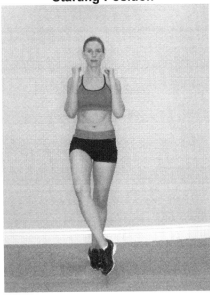

Execution

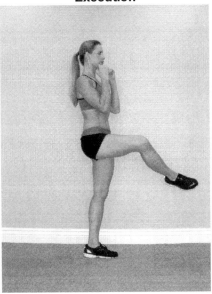

Starting Position: Stand in good posture with weight on the left foot with the knees slightly bent. Your hands should be held in front of your chest in two fists held next to your chin as a boxer, or placed together as if your were praying. Bend the right knee to 90 degrees and rotate the right leg outward at the hip, so the knee cap is pointed to the right and your heel is in front of your left ankle. The right foot should be about 6 inches off the ground in this position. Pull your shoulder blades down and back. Pull naval toward the spine. This is the starting position.

Execution: Exhale as you slowly raise the right leg using the adductor (the inner thigh muscle) without changing the knee angle. Inhale as you slowly lower the leg back to the starting position. Complete 10 reps and switch legs. Only lower the leg to a point where there is still tension in the inner thigh muscle.

> **Tips:** The only movement is the inner thigh muscle contracting. Do not move the knee joint or the rotation of the leg. The thigh muscle should have tension through the whole range of motion. Place one hand on a chair if your balance is unsteady.

Variations:

Pregnancy Modification: None needed. Place a sturdy chair on your right side to grab for balance.

Easier: Do sets of 7 on each leg. Place a sturdy chair on your right side to grab for balance.

Advanced: Do more sets. As pregnancy advances, the leg will become heavier. Do not use an ankle weight; it will change your posture.

Execution

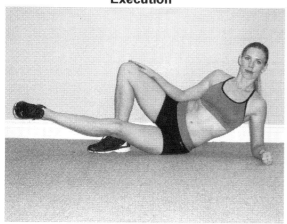

Starting Position: Lie on your left side and prop yourself up on your left elbow with your hand in a loose fist pointed forward. Try to hold your unsupported head in a neutral position. Bend your right knee and place your right foot flat on the ground behind your left knee. Press weight into the right foot. Left leg should be straight with the knee slightly bent and the foot in a neutral position. Pull naval toward the spine. Raise the left leg 2 inches off the ground. This is starting.

Execution: Exhale and use the inner thigh muscle to lift the left leg upwards a few inches. Inhale as you resist gravity and slowly lower the leg back to starting. The inner thigh should be tense through the whole motion, do not rest by setting the leg down. Perform 10 reps, then roll over to switch legs.

Tips: Your body will be inclined to roll backwards. You must make a conscious effort to keep the hips stacked. There is a tendency to let the body sag from the left shoulder; keep the torso supported so the spine is straight and not curved downward.

Variations:
You can also perform these while resting the left arm on a chair as pictured in the Oblique High Knee Variation. You will need to keep the left knee bent a bit to keep tension on the inner thigh muscle in this position.

Pregnancy Modification: None needed. As your belly gets larger you may want to lay along side a pillow and place your belly on top of it for support. It may be more comfortable for some (and nice when you feel tired) to fold up your left arm and lie your head on your left forearm on the ground. In this position, you may want to bring the legs further out in front of you by bending at the waist to maintain balance.

Advanced: Alternate leg sets with no rests for a continuous 60 reps. Perform sets of 20 reps. The leg will get heavier as pregnancy progresses. Ankle weights can create strain at the knee, so if you want to use them, lay them over the thigh just above the knees. The more weight you press into the right heel, the harder both inner thighs will work.

Side Chamber   **XXX**

Execution with Pregnancy Hand Position

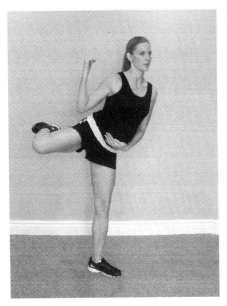

Starting Position: Stand upright and place all your weight on the left foot with the knee slightly bent. Rotate your left leg outward from the hip so that your left foot is pointed to 10 o' clock. Pull your shoulder blades down and back. Your hands should be in front of your chest in two fists held next to your chin as a boxer. The hips and shoulders should be squared forward and stay there throughout the move. Pull naval toward the spine.

Execution: In one coordinated motion: 1) Inhale as you bend slightly forward and lean your torso to the left at the waist while simultaneously using the right hip and right oblique muscle to lift the right leg out to the side bending the knee so the right foot is near the butt with pointed toes. Do not raise the knee any higher than you can raise your foot. The knee should be directed out to the side laterally, in-line with the hip and shoulder. Arms should adjust to the right, with the left fist near the right shoulder (pictured on facing page). **2)** Exhale as you focus on holding the leg in place by contracting the abs, right oblique and right hip muscle for 10 seconds. **3)** Resisting gravity, slowly reverse the motion and return to starting by taping the right foot back to the ground with total control (no gravity) and standing up straight. After 10 reps, switch legs.

Tips: Do not rotate the torso; keep the belly button pointed in the same direction. Do not rotate the right leg from the hip. That is, the right knee cap should be facing forward, not toward the ceiling. This move requires stretching. The stiffer your leg muscles are, the harder it will be to balance.

Variations:

Pregnancy Modification: Place a tall backed chair in front of you and place your hands just above the chair to grab when you need support. This is a great exercise to practice concentration and balance. It is very important that you keep the spine aligned while pregnant, twisting at the torso places too much stress on the back. There is no twisting in this move. During the third trimester the belly can have a weight of its own. I kept the right fist in boxing position, and the left arm wrapped softly under my belly. Switch the arms when you switch legs.

Easier: Place a tall backed chair in front of you and place your hands just above the chair to grab when you need support. You don't have to raise the leg as high as the picture. This is a great exercise to practice concentration and balance. Hold the chamber for 5 sec intervals.

Advanced: Stretch and practice so that your chamber leg is parallel to the floor and you can hold the position strongly for 60 sec. From the chamber position, perform a whip kick by keeping the entire body in the stationary chamber position, and simply extending the knee joint so that the right leg is completely straight, and then snap the foot back toward the butt. This is a speed kick.

Advanced Challenge: When you can successfully perform a whip kick without altering your body position from the chamber: Time how long you can perform continuous whip kicks before your form gives way (stop, never practice poor form). Next work on speed, by counting the number of kicks you can perform during that same time and try to fit more kicks into the time period. It is a great no-impact cardio exercise.

Execution Step 1

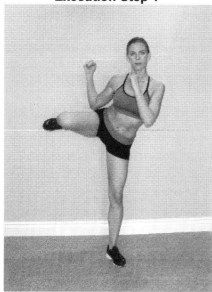

Execution Step 2

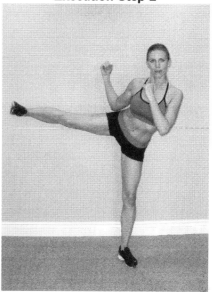

Starting Position: Stand upright in good posture with weight on the left foot and knee slightly bent. Pull your shoulder blades down and back. Your hands should be held in front of your chest in two fists held next to your chin as a boxer. Pull naval toward the spine.

Execution: 4 part move: 1) Inhale as you perform a side chamber, but this time the knee should be in front of you and the ankle should be next to the right hip. Pull your toes forward rather than pointing them. 2) Leading with the right heel, exhale as you forcefully extend the leg outwards laterally as if pushing someone. When the leg is fully extended the right oblique should be squeezing hard. 3) Pull the leg back into the chamber (Step 1). 4) Return to starting by taping the right foot back to the ground with total control (no gravity) and standing up straight. Perform 10 reps, then switch legs.

Tips: Do not rotate the torso; hips and shoulders should be squared forward. The knee cap should be facing forward, not up toward the ceiling. This move requires stretching. The stiffer your leg muscles are, the harder it will be to balance.

Variations:

Pregnancy Modification: None needed. Use a chair for support. This is a great exercise to practice concentration and balance. It is very important that you keep the spine aligned while pregnant, twisting at the torso places stress on the back. There is no twisting in this kick. During the third trimester the belly can have a weight of its own. I kept the right fist in boxing position and the left arm softly wrapped under my belly (shown in Side Chamber).

Easier: Place a tall backed chair in front of you and place your hands just above the chair to grab when you need support. You don't have to kick as high as the picture. Use the same technique to kick at knee height. This is a great exercise to practice concentration and balance. Practice holding the chamber for 5 second intervals.

Advanced: Perform 10 reps on each leg slowly and with total balance and control. Then perform 10 reps on each leg working on speed, balance and control for a cardio workout. The more upright you keep your torso, the harder you will work the oblique. If you have completely mastered form and control and have great balance, you can add a set of 20 where you alternate legs for each kick. Discontinue alternating during the third trimester.

Sea Saw Kicks

Starting Position

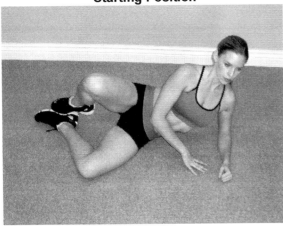

Execution First Kick

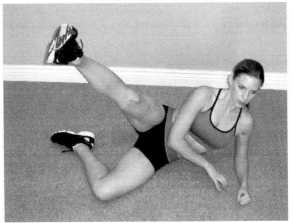

Starting Position: Lie on your left side and prop yourself up on your left elbow with your hand in a loose fist pointed forward. Try to hold your unsupported head in a neutral position. Place your right hand on the ground in front of your midsection. Shoulders and hips should be stacked. Bend your left knee keeping the leg on the ground. Rotate the right leg, and bend the right knee so the right knee is pointed upward 45 degrees and both feet are together. Pull naval toward the spine.

First Kick (This is a whip kick described under Advanced Side Chamber). Perform a whip kick by keeping the entire body in the stationary chamber position, and simply extending the knee joint so that the right leg is completely straight with the toes pointed toward the ceiling. Then snap the foot back toward the butt. The thigh and knee should remain exactly in the same place, only the lower leg should move. This is a speed kick, done with control, breathing the whole time. Perform 10 reps, and then move on to the second kick.

Execution Second Kick

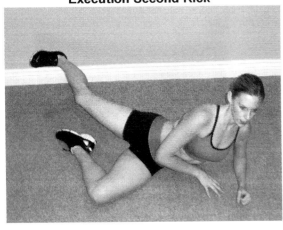

Second Kick This is a Standing Back Kick, performed while lying on the ground. You will now pull the toes forward, to lead with the heel. From the starting position, you will roll the torso forward so that you place some weight into the right hand. Cock the right leg, so that the ankle is now higher than the knee. Exhale as you extend the right leg backward and upward leading with the heel. You should get a solid glute squeeze and return to the starting position. Your body will rock forward and back a little, which is fine as long as the spine is straight and you are not twisting. This is a power kick, done with control, breathing the whole time. Perform 10 reps.

Tips: There is a tendency to let the body sag from the left shoulder; use the left shoulder muscles to support the torso so the spine is straight and not curved downward. This exercise works the right hip, so you must make a conscious effort to keep the hips stacked. Do not use ankle weights.

Variations:

Pregnancy Modification: None needed. Instead of placing the right arm on the ground in front of your belly, place your elbow on your waist and lay your forearm across the belly with your hand on your belly button. When you feel tired, it may be nice to do these while lying down. Fold up your left arm and lay your head on your left forearm on the ground. As your belly gets larger you may want to lay along side a pillow and place your belly on top of it for support. Perform the kicks as described.

Easier: Practice doing this move slowly and controlled. You should focus on feeling the muscles of the leg, hip and your abs. Do 5 reps of the first and second kick, then flip over and do the other leg.

Advanced: Perform 10 front kicks at rapid fire, followed by 10 powerful back kicks. Then, with no break, perform 20 kicks alternating between front and back. Your hips will burn and they are going to be sexy fabulous! Flip over and repeat on the other side.

Abductor Machine   XXX

Starting Position: Sit down in the machine and use the lever to adjust the foot pedals so that your knees are as close as they can be. Lock the lever and sit back into the seat. You will need to tilt your pelvis in order to press your lower back into the seat. If there is a head rest, use it.

Execution: Exhale and slowly spread your knees apart as far as you can using the hip muscle. This should be a slow and smooth motion. Inhale as you slowly resist the tension as the machine pushes your knees back together. The knees should not come crashing together; you must control the machine, not the other way around. Do not let the weight plates touch down. Repeat.

Tips: Be sure not to let the lower back lift off the seat by keeping the abs contracted. The hip muscle should never be resting during the whole set. Practice all the variations to keep the muscle guessing.

Variations:
Instead of using the machine, abduction can be done sitting, standing or lying down; see Easier, Advanced and Pregnancy modifications.

Pregnancy Modification: None needed. It may be nice, when you feel tired, to do these as a floor lying leg lift. Lie on your left side, folding up your left arm to lay your head on your left forearm on the ground. As your belly gets larger you may want to lay along side a pillow and place your belly on top of it for support. Lift the right leg up so that the foot is shoulder width apart; this is starting. Slowly raise the leg without rotating the knee cap (it should not turn toward the ceiling) until the hip muscle is squeezed; about one foot. Then, resisting gravity, slowly return to starting. Make sure your lower back remains relaxed. Your leg should be heavy enough, but if you want to use ankle weights, lay them over your thigh. If you can raise your leg higher, then your hips are not stacked.

Easier: Sit on a bench and place your hands on the outside of the knees and pushing inward as you try to spread your knees outward. This variation works the chest as well.

Advanced: Standing leg abduction isn't necessarily harder, but it does require balance. Get into good posture standing on one leg. Then focus on the hip muscle and use it to lift the leg straight out laterally from the body as high as you can, and then resist gravity as you return to starting. If you keep the hip bones parallel to the floor and maintain a pelvic tilt, you should only be able to lift the leg so that the toes are about 9 inches off the ground. Have something to grab onto for balance if needed. On the abductor machine, add more weight for each set.

Starting Position

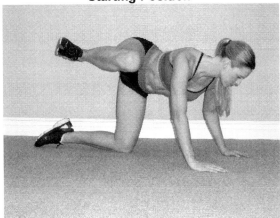

Execution

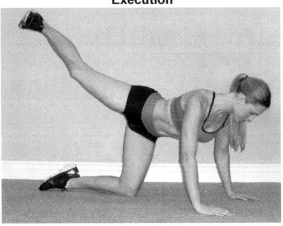

Starting Position: Get down on all fours. Lift your right leg outwards like a dog at a fire hydrant while keeping both hip bones pointed downward, parallel with the floor. Ideally, the knee and the ankle will be parallel to the floor. Bring the knee toward the arm pit and pull the toes forward so the heel will be leading. The foot will be perpendicular to the body and parallel to the floor.

Execution: Leading with the right heel, exhale as you forcefully extend the leg backwards and upwards as if pushing someone behind you. When the leg is fully extended the right glute should be squeezing hard and the foot should still be perpendicular to the body. Inhale as you bend the knee, pulling it back in toward the armpit. This is not a speed move, it is deliberate and forceful. Perform 10 reps, and then switch legs.

Tips: It is very easy to let the pelvis *open up* to the right, but you must keep the hip bones parallel to the floor to get any work out of the hip. You must keep your abs contracted so that your back does not sag downwards. This move requires stretching. The stiffer your leg muscles are, the harder it will be to get into the starting position. The exercise is effective even if you can't get your knee as high as the picture.

Variations:

Pregnancy Modification: None needed. However, you should discontinue this exercise when the weight of the belly and abdominal weakness can not support the lower back. It may help to get on all fours over a stack of pillows to rest your belly on. Decreasing the range of motion may allow you to continue these a little longer into the pregnancy.

Easier: Break it down. Stretch and practice holding the starting position until your hip is strong enough to lift your leg with the knee and ankle parallel to the floor. Once mastered, practice swinging your bent knee slowly from your armpit to behind you (without the kick) keeping the knee at the same height the whole range of motion. Practice the back kick by keeping the foot at the knee height rather than kicking upward like the picture (this should help keep your lower back straight). Then practice putting the steps together. Perform these in front of a wall or something, so that when you kick back you tap something with your heel so you remember to keep the toes pulled forward.

Advanced: In the starting position, place a stack of couch pillows under your knee as high as you can and still be able to clear it as your knee goes over them toward your armpit. As your hip muscle gets tired during a set, the leg will feel heavy and your knee will lower. If you don't work to keep your knee up, you will knock over the pillows. It serves as a motivator, but watch out - don't clear the pillows by cheating and *opening up* the pelvis.

Bench Press   **XXX**

Starting Position with Pregnancy Modification

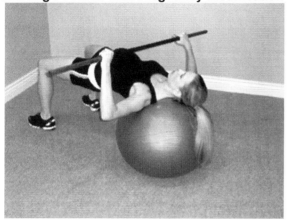

Execution with Pregnancy Modification

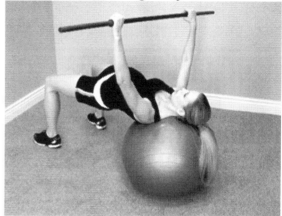

Starting Position: Lie on a bench with your knees bent and feet flat on the bench. Hold a straight bar over your chest with arms extended toward the ceiling. Wrists should be straight with your knuckles pointed toward the ceiling.

Execution: Inhale as you slowly lower the barbell until your upper arms are parallel to the floor. Your elbows should be directly below your wrists. Exhale as you push the barbell back to the starting position.

Tips: It is easier to keep your back flat if your feet are on the bench, rather than the floor. Draw navel to the spine, pressing the lower back into the bench. Keep the barbell directly over your nipples through the whole exercise. Do not lower your elbows below your shoulders; it strains the shoulder joint.

Variations:
You can use a curled bar if a straight bar is not available; just hold the bar wider than the curled section.

Easier: You don't have to use the big bench press station at the gym. Use a lighter weight bar or light weight dumbbells if the bar is too heavy. Do push ups until you are strong enough to handle a bar.

Pregnancy Modification: Do not attempt this modification until you have mastered a ball bridge. This technique should be used after week 20. Use a body ball instead of a bench. Sit on the ball while holding the bar. Walk your feet out letting the ball roll up your spine until it is under your upper back, and rest your head on it. Using your glutes and hamstrings, bridge upwards so that your body is parallel to the floor from your shoulders to your knees. Keep your knees directly over your ankles. Draw your navel in. Perform the bench press as described. The wider you spread your feet on the ground the more stability you will have.

Advanced: Perform the Pregnancy modification and make sure you are holding a strong bridge and pelvic tilt while performing each rep.

Dumbbell Flye

Starting Position with Pregnancy Modification

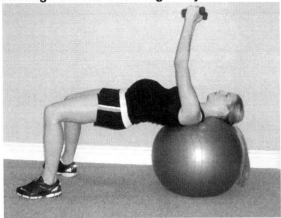

Execution with Pregnancy Modification

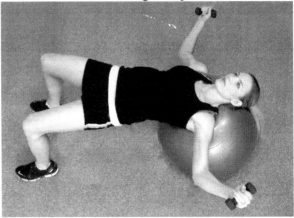

Starting Position: Lie on a bench with your knees bent and feet flat on the bench. Hold dumbbells over your chest with arms extended toward the ceiling and a slight bend in the elbow. Wrists should be directly over your shoulders (shoulder width apart) with your wrists straight. Palms should be facing each other. Dumbbells should be kept shoulder width apart.

Execution: Inhale and slowly bring the dumbbells outward and downward in a smooth arc until the chest muscles are stretched. The elbows should go slightly below the height of the shoulders, but the hands should not. Exhale and return the dumbbells through the same arc back to starting at shoulder width apart. The weights should not touch together.

Tips: The elbow joints should not change during the exercise; they should always be slightly bent pointed outward. My lower back looks arched, but it is an illusion. My butt is bigger and my belly is bigger, so it only looks like I am arching even though I am in a pelvic tilt.

Variations:

Easier: Use lighter dumbbells or water bottles.

Pregnancy Modification: Do not attempt this modification until you have mastered a ball bridge. This technique should be used after week 20. Use a body ball instead of a bench. Sit on the ball and walk your feet out letting the ball roll up your spine until it is under your upper back, and rest your head on it. Using your glutes and hamstrings, bridge upwards so that your body is parallel to the floor from your shoulders to your knees. The wider you spread your feet on the ground, the more stability you will have. Keep your knees directly over your ankles. Draw your navel in. Perform the pec flye as described.

Advanced: Perform the pregnancy modification and make sure you are holding a strong bridge and pelvic tilt while performing each rep.

Push Ups

Execution

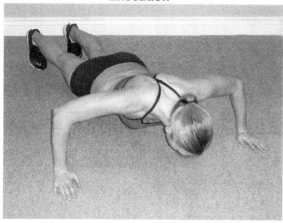

Starting Position: Get into a Plank-like position with your hands wide enough apart so that when you are in the down position, your wrists are directly below your elbows. Your weight should be equally balanced between your arms and feet. Your fingers should be pointed directly out in front of you.

Execution: Inhale and slowly lower yourself until your upper arms are parallel with the floor. Your elbows should be directly above your wrists. Exhale as you push back to the starting position.

Tips: Perform a pelvic tilt while doing a push up to prevent the lower back from sagging. Keep your head aligned with the spine.

Execution with Modification

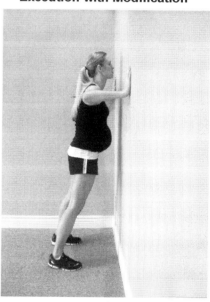

Variations:

Pregnancy Modification: Perform the Easier modifications. During the third trimester, do push ups against the wall. The closer your feet are to the wall, the easier it is.

Easier: The further your feet are apart the easier it is to balance. Do the push ups with your hands at an incline. Place hands on the edge of a bench, a step, a windowsill, a counter. Doing a push up on a bar may help if you get discomfort in the wrist because you can let you fingers curl over the edge. Perform push ups on the Smith Machine bar set to an appropriate height. You can also do push ups on the knees, but you must still keep the back flat.

Advanced: Do push ups with your feet together. Do push ups with your feet elevated on a step or book. The higher your feet, the more difficult it is. Do push ups with hands at different heights. Place one hand on a book and the other on the floor.

Advanced Balance Challenge: Place your hands on opposite sides of a Bosu with the flat side up, ball side down. Perform a push up. Setting your knees to the ground will make it easier. Performing a push up on a Bosu can help if you get discomfort in the wrist because you can let your fingers curl over the edge.

Burpy

Starting Position: Standing with good posture.

Execution: Bend at the waist and knees and place your hands on the ground at push up width apart. Jump feet backwards and get into plank position. Hold plank for 2 seconds. Jump feet back inwards and stand up.

Tips: Make sure you maintain abdominal contraction so your back does not sag downwards in the plank. After performing the move, stand up all the way into good posture before repeating the exercise. Head should be aligned with the spine throughout the exercise.

Variations:

Easier and Pregnancy Modification: When you place your hands on the ground, instead of jumping the feet backwards, use your hands to *walk* forward until you are in a plank. This takes the jarring motion out of the move and works your shoulders and chest more. Hold the plank and then walk your hands back and stand up. Discontinue when this exercise is no longer doable or your abs can't keep your back from sagging.

Advanced: Add a push up when in plank position. Add a jumping jack in the standing position. This move can be performed as a cardio speed drill or very slow and controlled. As your belly gets bigger, you can perform a burpy by walking your hands out into a plank, doing a push up, walking hands back, standing and slowly moving arms in an arc overhead to work the shoulders without doing the lower body portion of the jack. That is, keep the feet stationary for this part, so that you are not jumping.

Lateral Shoulder Raises   **XXX**

Starting Position

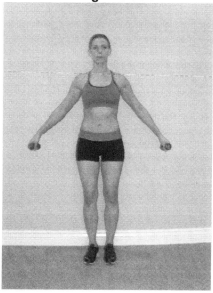

Execution

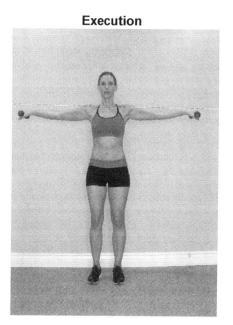

Starting Position: Stand with feet shoulder width apart, knees slightly bent. Place two very low weight dumbbells in each hand with palms facing inward. Wrists and elbows should be kept straight. Bring the abs to the spine. Start with the dumbbells far enough away from the body that there is tension in the shoulder muscles.

Execution: Exhale and slowly contract your shoulder muscles, raising your arms straight out to your sides. Stop rising when the arms are parallel with the floor. Then very slowly resist gravity as you lower the dumbbells as you inhale. Only lower the arms down to a point where there is still tension in the shoulders.

Tips: Pull the shoulder blades back and down to prevent your back and neck from getting involved. Hold the weights with a very loose grip. The tighter the grip, the more the arm muscles will help. If you still feel the muscles in the back of your neck, don't raise the arms as high as the execution picture. All fitness levels should use no more than two to three pound dumbbells. This will be difficult if you are not swinging your arms.

Variations:

Easier and Pregnancy Modification: Reduce the range of motion or perform this exercise while sitting in a chair and pressing the lower back flat. This reduces posture concerns. Use water bottles or no weight and you will still get an effective workout if you focus on the shoulder muscles.

Advanced: Do not use dumbbells heavier than 3 pounds. If it is easy, you are using momentum and your back, not your shoulder muscles. Do more sets or reps to make it harder. The slower you go, the harder it is.

Standing Up and Over

Execution

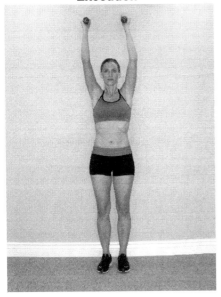

Starting Position: Same as Lateral Raise. Stand with feet shoulder width apart, knees slightly bent. Place two **very** low weight dumbbells in each hand with palms facing inward. Wrists and elbows should be kept straight. Bring the abs to the spine. Start with the dumbbells far enough away from the body that there is tension in the shoulder muscles.

Execution: Use your shoulder muscles to raise your arms straight out to your sides (Lateral Raise Execution). When the arms are parallel with the floor flip your hands over so the palms are facing the ceiling and continue to raise your arms in a large arc until you arms are overhead. Pictured on left. Then very slowly reverse through this motion resisting gravity. Only lower the arms down to a point where there is still tension in the shoulders. You will have to inhale and exhale several times through this motion.

Tips: Slow and controlled are the most important factors for this move. Keep your neck relaxed. If you feel your upper back or neck burning, do a few shoulder rolls then focus on the shoulder muscle doing the work. At the Execution pictured above, your arms should cover your ears. All fitness levels should use no more than two to three pound dumbbells. This will be difficult if you are not swinging your arms.

Variations:

Pregnancy Modification: You may want to perform this exercise while sitting in a chair and pressing the lower back flat. This eliminates posture concerns. Use water bottles or no weight and you will still get an effective workout if you focus on the shoulder muscles.

Easier: No one, except an experienced bodybuilder, should use more than 3 pounds for this move. Use water bottles instead of dumbbells or no weight at all. This move will fatigue the shoulders if done slowly enough with no weight.

Advanced: Do 3 sets of 10 reps. No one, except an experienced bodybuilder, should use more than 3 pounds for this exercise. If you can get through 3 sets of 10 without the shoulders burning, you are using momentum rather than your shoulder muscles to make the arc. The slower you go, the harder it is.

Starting Position   **Execution**

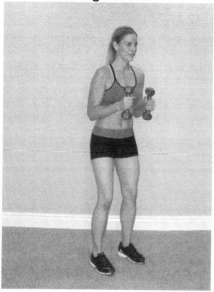

Starting Position: Stand with feet shoulder width apart, knees slightly bent. Waist should be bent with upper body slightly forward placing weight into the balls of feet. Place low weight dumbbells in each hand with palms facing inward. Wrists should be kept straight. Elbows should be bent and the angle should stay consistent though the move. Bring the abs to the spine. Start with the dumbbells far enough away from the body that there is tension in the shoulder muscles.

Execution: In one coordinated motion: 1) Exhale as you draw the elbows outward and up using the shoulder muscles. **2)** When the upper arms are parallel to the floor, rotate the shoulder joint to raise the forearms. Dumbbells will be higher than the shoulders and should still be inside the elbows. **3)** Inhale as you slowly return the dumbbells back to starting. You must keep the abs strong though the move to protect the back.

Tips: The only joint that moves is the shoulder. The hands and elbows change position, but the wrist and elbow joints do not move. Unless you are a bodybuilder, no one should use more than 10 pounds for this exercise. A person who uses 2 pounds dumbbells for a lateral raise could probably use 5 pound dumbbells for this exercise.

Variations:

Pregnancy Modification: This exercise requires that you are bent slightly forward at the waist, when your abs can no longer support your lower back, you will start to feel this exercise in your lower back. You should discontinue this exercise when you can't do it without engaging your lower back.

Advanced: Unless you are a bodybuilder, no one should use more than 10 pounds for this exercise. A person who uses 3 pounds for a lateral raise could probably use 5 to 8 pounds for this exercise. Shoulder exercises are more about technique than weight.

Seated Overhead Dumbbell Press

Starting Position

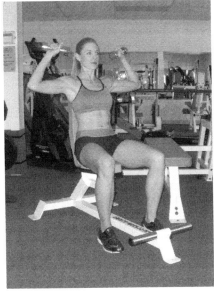

Execution

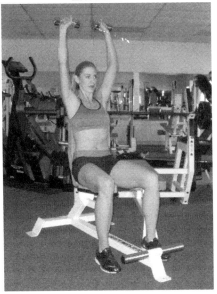

Starting Position: To protect your lower back, you must sit in a chair for this exercise. Sit in good posture with knees and toes aligned and pointed forward. Keep your head aligned with your spine and press your lower back into the chair by pulling your abs to the spine. Hold a dumbbell in each hand, palms facing forward with straight wrists, knuckles pointing toward the ceiling. Your upper arms should be parallel with the floor. Each wrist should be positioned between the shoulder and elbow.

Execution: Exhale as you press the dumbbells up and toward each other. At the top, the weights should come close to touching and your arms (elbows) should be almost fully extended. The elbow should be pointed outward through the movement. The path of the weights and elbows should follow an upside-down V overhead. Inhale as you slowly bend the elbows outward and downward until the dumbbells return to start with the upper arms parallel to the floor.

Tips: This gym chair has a foot bar. There is a tendency to push with the legs when using the foot bar which means using less core strength to keep good posture. Keep your feet flat on the floor, with ankles under the knees. If you feel yourself pushing into your feet, the dumbbells are too heavy. If you feel your lower back arching off the chair, you are using too much weight. Keep your abs tight and lower back pressed into the chair.

Variations:

Pregnancy Modification: You will need to decrease the weight as pregnancy progresses.

Advanced: Unless you are a bodybuilder, no one should use more than 12 pounds for this exercise.

Caution! The shoulder is a delicate joint, with many tiny muscle fibers. It is one of the most commonly over worked joints in the body. People often use too much weight for shoulder exercises, so pick something light, do it right and add another set if you need a challenge.

Seated Overhead Triceps Extension   **XXX**

Starting Position
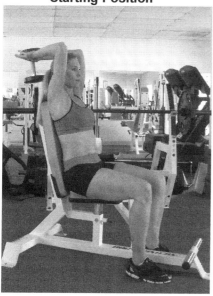

Execution
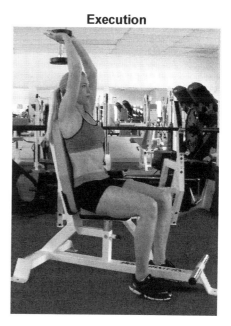

Starting Position: You must sit in a chair for this exercise to protect your lower back. Sit in good posture with knees and toes aligned and pointed forward. Keep your head aligned with your spine and press your lower back into the chair by pulling your abs to the spine. Hold a dumbbell behind your head with both hands, by interlocking the thumbs around one end, palms facing flat toward the ceiling. The upper arms should be back, covering the ears and the elbows should be facing forward, just like the knees.

Execution: Without moving the upper arms, exhale as you press the dumbbell upwards toward the ceiling until the arms are almost fully extended. The wrists can be bent backward at the top. Inhale as you slowly allow gravity to lower the dumbbell back down to starting position. Your triceps should feel stretched, not resting.

Tips: As your triceps get tired the elbows will drift outward and forward. Keep the arms close to your ears. Don't bow your head forward.

Variations:

Pregnancy Modification: You must sit in a chair to do this exercise to protect your lower back. If you feel your lower back arching away from the chair even though you are doing a pelvic tilt, the weight is too heavy and you will need a lighter dumbbell.

Advanced: Finish one set of ten, and then without breaking, switch to a dumbbell that is half the weight and perform single arm triceps extension, doing 10 reps with each arm. This is one set, break and repeat.

Triceps Dip

**Advanced Starting Position &
Easier or Pregnancy Execution**

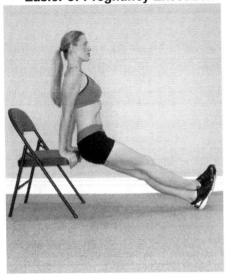

Starting Position: Sit on the edge of a bench. Slide your hands, palms down, just under your hips with your fingers hanging down the front side of the seat. Your elbows should be pointed directly back from the shoulders, not outward. Extend your feet out in front of you so that your butt is off the bench, but fairly close. Legs should be extended with heels on the ground, but the knees should not be locked. Most of your body weight should be in your triceps (back of upper arm) with the elbows slightly bent.

Execution: Slowly lower your body until your upper arms are about parallel with the floor. Your hips should drop straight down. Exhale as you push through your arms, to lift your body back to starting. Your back should stay within an inch or two of the bench the whole time.

Tips: Do not use your legs to help; you will end up lifting your pelvis out of alignment with the spine. If you feel there is a lot of tension in your shoulders, you may be dipping down too low. Bend your knees and place feet flat on the floor to take tension off the shoulders.

Advanced Challenge

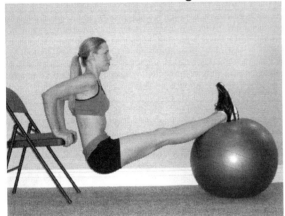

Easier Execution

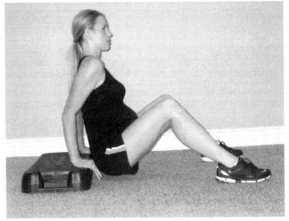

Variations:

Pregnancy Modification: None needed. You will need to reduce the range of motion or spread the legs to accommodate your belly. Holding the starting position also works the triceps. Or perform the Easier modification.
Easier: To make the first picture easier, bend your knees and place feet flat on the ground. This allows the legs to help the triceps lift the body. Or practice holding the starting position without the dip. Or do a dip with a smaller range of motion; you can use a step instead of a bench, so the dip is very small and your feet are not at such a great angle from your hips.
Advanced: Get into the starting position. Now pull the shoulder blades back and down; you will need to angle your hands outward from the hips. This helps keep the elbows directly behind the shoulders. You can also cross your ankles so that only one heel is in contact with the ground or elevate your ankles by placing them on a step or bench.
Advanced Challenge: While sitting on a bench, extend legs and place both heels on a body ball. The closer your feet are together the more you will have to use your core to keep your balance. With your heels on the ball, roll slightly forward so your butt is just off the bench. Hold this position for 10 seconds. Pull back to sitting on the bench. If you are stable enough and strong enough, do 3 sets of dips with feet on the ball. Discontinue during the second trimester.

Skull Crusher

Starting Position with Pregnancy Modification

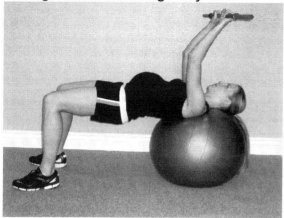

Execution with Pregnancy Modification

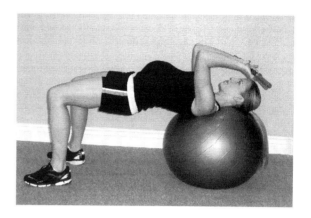

Starting Position: Lie on a bench with your knees bent, feet flat on the bench. With extended arms, hold a bar directly over your shoulders, palms facing your feet. Wrists should be straight and directly over your shoulders with your knuckles pointed toward the ceiling. Now bend your elbows, without moving your upper arms, until you feel tension in the triceps. This is the starting position.

Execution: Keep upper arms and elbows stationary. As you inhale, bend your elbows and slowly allow gravity to lower the bar towards your hairline. Elbows should be pointing toward the ceiling. Then exhale as you simultaneously draw the naval to the spine and use only the triceps to push the bar back to the starting position.

Tips: People tend to allow their elbows to migrate outward from each other. This makes the exercise ineffective. Keep the elbows stationary and directly over the shoulder. Keep your back flat on the bench, by drawing the navel to the spine.

Variations:

Pregnancy Modification: Do not attempt this modification until you have mastered a ball bridge. After week 20 you should not lie on your back for extended time, so move the skull crusher onto a body ball. Get into the starting position by sitting on a body ball while holding the bar; then slowly walk your feet forward as you roll the ball up your spine until it is under your shoulders and head. Be sure to bridge your pelvis upwards until your body is parallel with the floor from head to knee. The wider you spread your feet on the ground, the more stability you will have. Knees should be directly over the ankles. Perform the skull crusher as described. The EZ curl bar weighs 25 lbs. Use a weighted straight bar (6-15 lbs.) if you need lower weight. If you do these slowly enough, even 6 lbs. will be a good workout.

Easier: Use a very light weight bar or a closet dowel.

Advanced: The Pregnancy modification can be tough. If you bridge hard through an entire set your butt is going to burn.

Cable Rope Triceps Extension

Starting Position

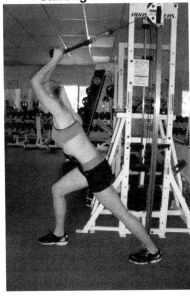

Execution

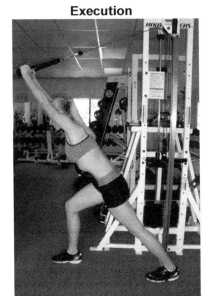

Starting Position: Attach a rope to the high-pulley cable machine and grasp the ends with your pinkie fingers against the balls at the end of the rope. Bring your arms overhead and turn your back to the machine. Assume a wide stride stance. Knees should be slightly bent and the heel closest to the machine can be off the floor. Your upper arms should cover your ears and your body should be straight from elbows to the back heel. Draw the navel to the spine.

Execution: Exhale as you extend your forearms until your elbows are extended. Your upper arms and elbows should stay locked in one place. Your body will be straight from hands to back heel. Inhale as you slowly allow the machine tension to draw your hands back to the starting position.

Tips: Keep your back flat by drawing the abs in. Don't drop your head down, keep it aligned with the spine.

Variations: This can also be performed by wrapping a resistance band around something taller than you.

Pregnancy Modification: As your waistline gets larger, you will have to bear more weight on the front foot in order to protect your back. Remember the tension is pulling you backwards, so if you lean forward more, and bear more weight on the front foot, gravity will assist you in keeping proper back alignment. This modification will not decrease the effectiveness of the exercise.

Easier: If you can't seem to get into this position, stand upright with feet parallel and shoulder width apart. Turn your back to the cable machine and align your upper arms so they are parallel with the floor and your hands are by your ears. From this starting position, the motion of extending the lower arms is the same. This is easier because your upper arms don't have to stretch back by your ears, however this position doesn't protect your back as much. If you feel pulling in the low back, sit a little more into your stance and do a stronger pelvic tilt.

Standing Dumbbell Bicep Curl   XXX

Starting Position Pregnancy Modification   **Execution**

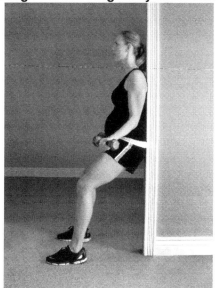 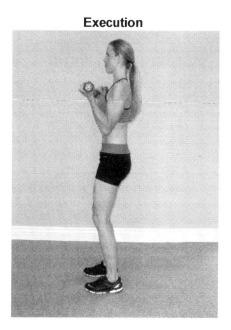

Starting Position: Stand with feet shoulder width apart holding a dumbbell in each hand. Pull your shoulder blades down and together to hold your posture. Wrists should be straight and arms pronated so your palms are facing forward. Place your elbows against your waist just in front of your shirt seam. Biceps will have tension in this position.

Execution: Keeping your elbows stationary, exhale as you bend your elbows and curl the dumbbells up towards your shoulders while drawing the naval to the spine. Curl the dumbbells about three quarters of the way to the shoulder. Inhale as you slowly allow gravity to lower the dumbbells back to starting position without releasing tension in the biceps.

Tips: Keep your back straight, head aligned with the spine. Do not curl your wrists; your knuckles should be aligned with your forearm though the whole move. If you feel your torso swaying as you curl, you are lifting too fast or using too much weight...get rid of the momentum that is causing your body to move.

Variations:

Advanced: Alternate each arm curl rather than doing both arms at the same time. This challenges your balance and back stabilizing muscles more.

Second & Third Trimester Variations:
As your stomach enlarges, your center of gravity will move forward. This will cause your back to overcompensate. I suggest backing up to the vertical bar of a Smith Machine, so that the bar is between your shoulder blades. Push your back flat against the bar, bending your knees as much as needed. Feet should be wider than shoulder width apart. Perform the curl as described. If you are not at a gym, any vertical bar will work. If you are at home, fit your shoulder blades on either side of a door jam, or just back up to a wall. Having a support between the shoulder blades is better because it opens up the chest. Leaning against a wall is better than just standing, but the wall will push your shoulders forward more, putting less tension on the biceps. You will probably need to decrease the weight as pregnancy advances.

Hammer Curl

Starting Position

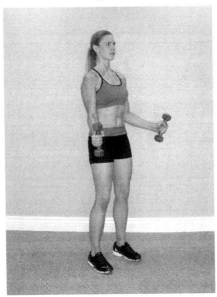

Starting Position: Stand, feet shoulder width apart in good posture with a slight bend in the knees and hips. Hold a dumbbell in each hand with palms facing your sides. Pull your shoulder blades down and together; this will angle your arms outward. Place your elbows against your waist. Wrists should be straight through the whole move. Draw navel to the spine.

Execution: Keeping your elbows stationary, exhale as you bend your elbows and curl the dumbbell up towards your shoulder. Curl the dumbbells about three quarters of the way to your shoulders. Inhale as you slowly allow gravity to lower the dumbbells back to starting position without releasing tension in the biceps.

Tips: Keep your back straight, head aligned with the spine. Make sure your shoulders are not shrugging upwards. Drawing the shoulder blades together really supports posture.

Variations:

Second & Third Trimester Variations:
As your stomach enlarges, your center of gravity will move forward. This will cause your back to overcompensate. You can sit in a chair, but you will need to press your lower back into the chair, which may be difficult to control unless there is a foot bar for your feet to push on. At home, place the chair in front of a wall, so you can press the balls of your feet into the wall to push your lower back into the chair. I suggest standing and backing up into the vertical bar of a Smith Machine, so that the bar is between your shoulder blades. If you are not at a gym, any vertical bar will work. If you are at home, fit your shoulder blades on either side of a door jam, pictured in Standing Dumbbell Biceps Curl. Having a support between the shoulder blades is better because it opens up the chest more. Leaning against a wall is better than just standing, but the wall will push your shoulders forward more putting less tension on the biceps. You can also sit on an incline bench set at a slight recline. Let your arms dangle naturally from your shoulders. The dumbbells will be behind you in this starting position. You will probably need to decrease the weight as pregnancy advances. Perform this exercise with water bottles if that is all the weight you can manage.

Advanced: Once you master this move, rather than getting heavier dumbbells, perform this exercise on an incline bench. When you are reclined, your elbows will be hanging down behind you. This isolates the bicep and makes it harder. Another way to make it more challenging is to hold the dumbbells at one end rather than the middle. The uneven load is harder to lift.

Concentration Curl

Starting Position

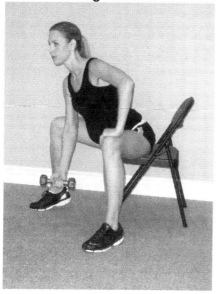

Execution

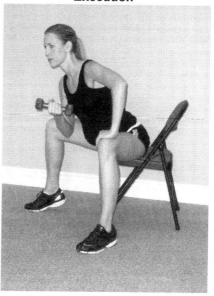

Starting Position: Sit on a bench or chair straddling one corner. Legs spread wide with knees stacked on top of ankles. Place a dumbbell in the right hand. With a straight back, lean forward from the waist and place your right elbow against the inside of your right thigh just above your knee. The dumbbell should be hanging near the inside of your right ankle. Raise the right heel off the floor so you don't have to bend over so far. Place the left hand on top of the left thigh with the left elbow pointed outward away from the body to support the back. Bring the abs to the spine so that the back does not sag downward. Slightly bend the right elbow so there is tension in the biceps. This is the starting position.

Execution: Exhale as you draw the dumbbell in an arc up toward your shoulder. The dumbbell should come within an inch of your collar bone; squeeze the bicep muscle. Inhale as you slowly resist gravity, stretching the bicep muscle back to the starting position without releasing tension in the biceps.

Tips: Keep your back straight, head aligned with the spine. Keep the shoulders parallel with the floor; you don't want to rotate at the waist. If you find yourself leaning back in order to lift the weight, the weight is too heavy. Keep the wrist straight; don't curl it toward your body.

Variations:

Pregnancy Modification: None needed. This position isolates the bicep, thereby taking strain off the back and shoulders making it a good exercise for advanced maternity. You will need to use lighter dumbbells as pregnancy progresses.

Easier: Use lower weight to make it easier.

Advanced: This position isolates the bicep, thereby taking strain off the back and shoulders, so you can challenge yourself with more weight without worrying about injuring yourself. In this position, you can also *spot* yourself by using your free hand to assist the dumbbell when the rep gets hard.

Twenty-Ones

Starting Position	Execution Step 2	Pregnancy Modification Execution Step 3

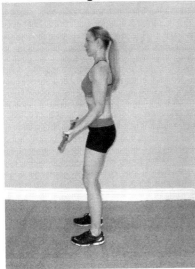 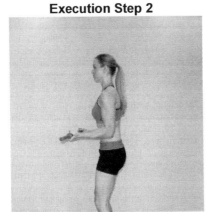 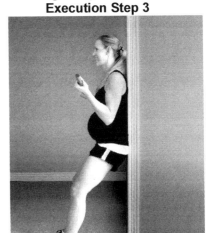

Starting Position: Stand, feet shoulder width apart holding a flat or curl bar. Keep your elbows at the seam of your shirt and close to your sides at all times. Pull your shoulder blades down and together. Draw the naval to the spine. Curl the bar away from the legs until there is tension in the biceps.

Execution: This exercise is one set of 21 reps. The 21 reps break down into 3 sets of 7 reps done with no break. Exhale as you bend your elbows and curl the bar to waist height (Step 2). Your elbows should be at a 90 degree angle. Slowly inhale as you resist gravity and slowly lower the bar to the starting position. Your bicep should feel stretched and have tension. Perform 7 reps. Then beginning at waist height (Step 2), curl the bar up towards your shoulders as you exhale (Step 3). Inhale as you resist gravity and slowly lower the bar no lower than waist height (Step 2). Perform 7 reps. Finally, perform a whole biceps curl from starting position to Step 3 as you exhale. Inhale as you slowly allow gravity to lower the bar back to starting position. Perform 7 reps to complete one set of 21 reps.

> **Tips:** Keep your back straight, head aligned with the spine. Draw navel to the spine. Do not curl your wrists; your knuckles should be aligned with your forearm.

Second & Third Trimester Variations:
As your stomach enlarges, your center of gravity will move forward. This will cause your back to overcompensate. I suggest backing up to the vertical bar of a Smith Machine, so that the bar is between your shoulder blades. Push your back flat against the bar, bending your knees as much as needed. Feet should be wider than shoulder width apart with knees bent. Perform the curl as described. If you are not at a gym, any vertical pole will work. If you are at home, fit your shoulder blades on either side of a door jam. Having a support between the shoulder blades opens up the chest and protects the lower back. You will need to use a lighter bar as pregnancy progresses.

Calf Raises   **XXX**

Starting Position: Stand in good posture with the knees and hips slightly bent, feet shoulder width apart. Toes should be pointed straight ahead. Your hands should be held in front of your chest in two fists held next to your chin as a boxer, or placed together as if you were praying. Pull naval toward the spine.

Execution: Exhale as you press your weight into the balls of your feet and lift your heels as high as you can. Inhale as you slowly lower heels down to starting. Try not to transfer weight to the heels.

Tips: If you lose your balance, don't flail your arms. Instead, contract your abs harder. Balance is in the core. Balance takes concentration and abdominal visualization.

Variations:

Pregnancy Modification: None needed. Place a high backed chair in front of you to help with balance.

Easier: Perform near a chair or something sturdy to grab onto if you lose your balance.

Advanced: Place balls of feet on edge of a step, a curb, or on two small weight plates so your heels are hanging off. Do 10 reps. Then, immediately angle toes outward in a ballet plie position and complete 10 reps. Then immediately point toes inward (pigeon toed) and do 10 more reps to complete 1 set. Do not add dumbbells, practicing balance is more important.

Advanced Challenge: Perform calf raises with the balls of your feet on 2.5 lb. weight plates. Do 10 reps very slowly. As you come down, try to touch your heels all the way to the ground without transferring weight to the heels. Then do 20 calf raises very quickly with a small range of motion, followed by 10 more done slowly.

One Leg Calf Raise   **XXX**

Starting Position: Stand on your right foot, placing your weight on the ball of the foot. Cross the left leg behind the right, wrapping the left foot around the right ankle. Stand in good posture with knees and hips slightly bent. Your hands should be held in front of your chest in two fists held next to your chin as a boxer, or placed together as if your were praying. Pull your shoulder blades down and back. Pull naval toward the spine.

Execution: Exhale as you press your weight into the ball of your foot and lift your heel as high as you can. Inhale as you slowly lower it down to starting.

Tips: Keep your abs tight, balance is in the core. The harder you contract and focus on the core the more stable your body will be.

Variations:

Pregnancy Modification: None needed. Stand next to a wall or a tall backed chair and place one hand on it.

Easier: Stand next to a wall and place one hand on it. Practice standing on one foot. Then practice balancing on the ball of one foot. When your balance improves, add the calf raise.

Advanced: Do not place any weight in the heel during the set.

Chapter 15

Postpartum Recovery

Don't wait until after delivery to read this chapter!

I hope you are reading this chapter before you deliver, so that you know what to do before you get too busy to pick up a book. If not, congratulations on the arrival of your baby! I hope you, your baby and family are healthy and happy. Enjoy as much of this time as you can. Now, back to business! If you have been following this program up until delivery day you have already started your postpartum recovery. By maintaining abdominal muscle tone and a strong metabolism you are well on your way. If you had a vaginal delivery with no episiotomy, tears or other physical complications, recovery to your best body ever should be a smooth-ish road. If you stopped exercising at some point or had an episiotomy, vaginal tear or a C-section, your recovery is going to take longer.

So the caterpillar has finished a nine month incubation
and is now a tiny butterfly in the outside world....
you finally have your body all to yourself again.
It's time to claim the Mommy Fabulous figure you worked nine months for.

I heard you shouldn't start exercising until six weeks postpartum, is that true?

This is not true. If you had a vaginal delivery with no episiotomy or tears the American College of Obstetric and Gynecology guidelines state: "Physical activity can thus be resumed as soon as physically and medically safe. This will certainly vary from one woman to another, with some being capable of engaging in an exercise routine within days of delivery. There are no published studies to indicate that, in the absence of medical complications, rapid resumption of activities will result in adverse effects." [56]
While there are no known complications with returning to training, the ACOG wisely recommends that you gradually resume activities. Just because you are no longer pregnant, doesn't mean you are fit enough for sprints three days postpartum. I will guide you through a safe and gradual recovery program that will deliver rapid results by working smart, not necessarily hard. You absolutely can and should continue to exercise with a program that is considerate of your healing wounds. There is no reason you should get out of shape over the next six weeks.
You will have a postpartum check up at around six weeks post delivery. The reasons for this visit include making sure any tears or episiotomies have healed, making sure your uterus has shrunk back to pear size, giving you the green light for sex and tampons, discussing birth control, to see how you are coping with motherhood and to answer any questions you have. This visit is not to assess whether you can walk, run, jump or catch a ball. Many people assume this last check up is intended to give you clearance to resume your normal activities, but it has very little to do with your fitness capabilities.

What's the rush? Can't I take it slowly and get into shape over the next year or two?

You need to do what you are comfortable with and what will make you happy. Think about postpartum recovery this way; if you break your arm, are you going to wait six weeks, six months or a year to start rehabilitating the injury? By that time the bone will have grown back together, possibly not straight, scar tissue will have formed and the muscles will have atrophied. Now that the injury has repaired itself into a new and unfortunate position, you want to gain your old functionality back? That makes no sense. You have just had a major abdominal trauma. You need to ensure that the abdominal muscles heal into a state that you want. I'm not suggesting that if a woman does nothing for a year after she has a baby she will never be able to have a great looking stomach. I am saying it is a lot easier to shape a healing wound than to try to remold an old wound that has set itself.

I hate to say it, but this is the easy part. I am more tired now that Talia is two years old than I was two days postpartum. Seriously, my husband can vouch. The baby is stationary. You sleep when they sleep, you are on leave from work, you *do* have the time. It is about priorities. You are a priority. You have got eight to ten months max before things get really busy. Life is only going to get busier, more complicated and your baby is only going to get heavier. Don't wait until you can't keep up with a mobile toddler!

Three Elements to a Mommy Fabulous Figure

Exercise

Fitness is just as important now as it was while you were pregnant. I know you are busy, and tired, but your health is not a last priority. Exercise is proven to elevate mood. Postpartum depression is not a choice. You have had nine months of pregnancy hormones running through your system that will now come crashing down. I can say that exercise is what kept me sane after I delivered. You need a break from your new 24-7 job, motherhood. You are on sleeping duty when baby is sleeping, so this doesn't count as a break. Every single day you need time to unwind, decompress and let go of the stresses of motherhood. This time should be spent exercising. Lying around watching TV doesn't help release any tension nor does it allow you to focus on yourself. Ideally, I think you should go to the gym. Getting out of the house and away from your baby will allow you to focus on yourself. Remember that you are still you, not just someone's mother.

As for postpartum resumption of activities, the ACOG recommendations note that rapid resumption has no adverse effects, but gradual return to former activities is advised. During the first six weeks postpartum your abdomen and pelvic floor are healing, so you don't want to do activities that will put pressure on them. The faster you can regain tone in your pelvic floor the better. The postpartum plan includes many suggestions for incorporating recovery techniques into daily life with a newborn. You will basically continue the Mommy Fabulous Program only in reverse and with a new timeline. I have outlined activities and time suggestions to help you decide what is appropriate and reasonable for a fitness recovery. Listen to your body and use your own judgment. Consistency is key! If you follow the Mommy Fabulous Program everyday, you will look better than ever in four to six months.

Diastasis Recti

Check to see if you developed abdominal muscle separation, a large proportion of women do. Page 102 will show you how to do this. Don't make this condition worse by exercising without addressing the problem. Try to help your abdomen heal correctly during the first six weeks postpartum by doing the exercise described on page 102. You may want to get additional help with this.

Food

Continue eating Mommy Fabulous style. Healthy eating habits, which I hope you have formed, are a lifestyle. You don't have to follow Chapter One anymore. Since you are not pregnant you can enjoy sushi again. Don't change your dietary habits as you are going to need the energy and *Clean Burning Fuel* is the best fuel to encourage weight loss. If you follow my nutrition advice, you don't have to worry about dieting. When you eat Mommy Fabulous style you will find that your body will really only be interested in what it needs. Continue eating three meals and two snacks daily, just make the portions smaller. Keeping blood sugar level will prevent you from overeating at meals.

Don't you dare go back to caffeine and sugar! They will sabotage your postpartum weight loss like they would have sabotaged your pregnancy weight gain. Caffeine is a particularly bad idea. When you turn to caffeine for energy postpartum, you will just end up hooked and more tired overall because caffeine interferes with restful sleep. Likewise, alcohol will ruin your metabolism and encourages belly fat retention.

Nursing Mothers

If you are nursing, you should continue eating Mommy Fabulous style, but you may need to make your snacks more substantial to keep up with the calorie demands of breastfeeding and exercising. *Clean Burning Fuel* will ensure you are not transferring chemicals to your precious baby through breast milk. Caffeine can create problems for the nursing mother. Not only will caffeine interfere with you getting restful sleep, but it may make your baby more cranky and unable to sleep, which will in turn make you more tired. Caffeine is a diuretic, so it may interfere with your milk production. Moderate weight loss and exercise will not interfere with nursing.[62] If you find your baby is not gaining weight, you may not be producing enough milk. This generally has more to do with not drinking enough fluids or eating enough calories than with maternal weight loss. You may want to nurse or pump before exercising for more breast comfort. Make sure you wear a good supportive bra to exercise in.

Posture

I can not express how much your postpartum posture will affect how well your abs recover from pregnancy. Heavy breasts will have you hunched forward with your back curved and your poor empty belly sagging outward relaxed. Plus, you will be doing a lot of forward lifting, holding, diapering and bathing. Even if you didn't get backaches during pregnancy, you could start getting them now. While pregnant you had the luxury of having a backache, now your baby will not take back pain for an answer. Your upper back and abs should support your posture. You must consciously make your abs hold your pelvis in alignment. Apply the Body English principals from Chapter 12 during daily activities. Proper posture may be more challenging now that the baby is on the outside.

Episiotomies, Tears, Cesarean Sections and Fitness

If you had an episiotomy or tears, your recovery will take longer. Your wound should be healed in two to four weeks, but the area may be sore or painful for four to six weeks postpartum. You want to avoid exercises that put pressure on your wound, such as heavy lifting, and you want to avoid activities that might open the tear, like kicking. Kegels and pelvic tilts can help the healing process; do three sets of ten every day. Add any of the suggestions from the Sample Postpartum Recovery Program below that do not cause pain. After the stitches have healed you can begin training more aggressively.

Cesarean section is a major surgery. After a C-section, the pelvic floor doesn't have much healing to do aside from being relieved of the pressure from the baby and placenta. However, your abdominal muscles were stretched during pregnancy and then cut for the delivery. Begin with Kegels and any of the below suggestions that do not cause pain. A C-section should be healed in four to five weeks postpartum. Your muscles can then be strengthened in the same way as if you had a vaginal delivery unless your doctor says otherwise. It will take deep concentration to regain control of the injured muscles.

Sample Postpartum Recovery Program
for a vaginal delivery with no episiotomy, tears or other physical complications

The first four to six weeks postpartum are a time of physical healing. Some women will experience little perineal soreness while others may experience a lot of soreness that lasts longer. Exercise resumption should be done at an individualized pace. Below, you will find suggestions to get you started. Do what you are comfortable with and adjust your personal timeline accordingly.

Twenty-Four Hours Postpartum

Twenty-four hours after delivery, begin doing pelvic tilts and Kegels as often as you can while in your hospital bed. A good regimen would be: four tilts every three hours and four Kegels every three hours. Or ten tilts and Kegels three times per day. Most women with uncomplicated vaginal deliveries stay in the hospital two nights. Sleep as much as you can.

3 Days Postpartum
Add these activities:

- When you return home on day three postpartum, try to wear a Bella Band (available at most maternity stores or online) for three hours at a time. It works like a torso cast or flexible girdle and serves as a reminder to use your ab muscles during daily activities. Through the Mommy Fabulous Fitness Program you have maintained abdominal muscle tone, which means that your abs *remember* that they are supposed to hold tight. However, without the baby inside, they are stretched out too far to hold tight. You must constantly remind them where they should be, and they will quickly *remember*. The longer you wait to remind them where they should be, the more they will *forget* what tight is like and you will end up having to retrain them later- much harder than reminding them now.

- Constantly correct your posture! Keep your shoulders and abs pulled back. It is easy to let the shoulders roll forward and push the abs out as you curl your body over your baby. The Mommy Fabulous abdominal visualization concept from Chapter 11 is still applicable, only now the baby is on the outside of your abdomen. When you are holding your baby, and feel the baby's body touching your stomach, draw your naval to your spine. There is a tendency to push the abdomen outwards when something is touching it, which is definitely NOT where you want your stomach to be going. The small bundle of joy is still an abdominal reminder.

- While breastfeeding, pumping or bottle feeding sit upright in your rocking chair, glider or sofa and draw your naval toward your spine pressing your lower back into the chair, exhaling and holding for five to ten seconds. Repeat continuously. Halfway through feedings switch to this exercise: spread your knees to hip width apart. Pretend you are trying to squeeze your knees together, but there are invisible hands trying to pry them apart. You are basically making your adductor muscles fight your abductors. Hold the tug of war for ten seconds; repeat continuously. Another seated, low intensity exercise is to sit upright in a chair with legs together, and ankles under the knees. Wrap baby in a blanket and lay the baby on your lap parallel with your thighs. Perform calf raises until your caves burn, then set the heels on the ground and lift the balls of your feet for toe taps until your shins burn. Babies enjoy this soft bouncing.

161

- The rocking chair is comfortable, maybe too comfortable. Try limiting its use to nighttime. During the day sit on a body ball while holding your baby and lean back into a pelvic tilt.

- Sleep whenever the baby sleeps. I'm serious about this. Well rested people have a much easier time losing weight; it is well documented scientifically. Sleep also has a great affect on mood. Even modest sleep deprivation can leave you feeling sad and with little energy to exercise. Remember that exercise releases endorphins which make people feel happier. Sleep and exercise together will do wonders to help you mentally and physically get through the hard weeks ahead. Your body also does its most productive healing during sleep. Lots of sleep is part of the recovery program.

- Go out for walks. Yes four day old babies can be outside or in a mall if it is raining. You took the baby outside to get home from the hospital, right? Just don't let anyone near the baby. Stand up straight and hold your abs tight.

- As far as exercise is concerned, you mainly want to avoid activities and exercises that create abdominal cavity pressure because the force will bear down on your healing pelvic floor. Exercises that cause too much pelvic floor pressure at this time are crunches, any weightlifting done overhead, activities that including bouncing or jumping. Examples of exercises that do not create abdominal cavity force include Kegels, pelvic tilts, the Floor Work Exercises (page 101) and walking. Exercises can wait until day 7.

- Do Kegels as much as you can; your future urinary and sexual health depend on a strong pelvic floor.

7 Days Postpartum
Add these activities:

- Time to return to the gym (or the home gym). I encourage you to get out of the house and away from your baby for one hour a day. You need a one hour break from your new responsibilities everyday. Exercise elevates the mood. Working out helped me through the hard transition to motherhood and lifted the baby blues. Remember all the concentration and focus the Mommy Fabulous exercises took? Well you need to keep practicing the method, and it may be difficult to concentrate at home with all the chores, a baby and gear to assemble. Walk casually on the treadmill, go lightly on the elliptical, stretch, any Mommy Fabulous exercises that do NOT involve weights are a good idea. Perform exercises slowly. If you feel like you are bearing down on your pelvic floor, discontinue the exercise you are doing until the pelvic floor muscles gain more tone.

- Decrease the intensity of the activities you are doing if you notice an increase in the amount of bleeding. It may be a sign that you are overdoing it. Once you have fully stopped bleeding, between week one and week six postpartum you can start more aggressive training.

- There is no real reason to get on a scale. Mommy Fabulous is not focused on numbers; focus on how you look and feel. My goal for you is a better body, not your old body, so I really don't care to shoot for getting your old weight back.

- You are not allowed to use the back rest on a chair until you are satisfied with your abs.

162

This may take four months or much longer depending on how high you are making your fitness a priority. At dinner, at the computer, you must remind your abs to work not sag. Sit on a body ball.

- Sleep every time that baby does! I don't care if the laundry never gets folded and you live out of the dryer or if your house is a mess. You need a lot of sleep to have energy to workout. You need to prioritize. Believe me, neither you nor your husband, are going to remember that the house was dirty for two months of your lives, even if it does cause tension today. If he wants dinner and a clean house he can do it himself. I am sure that if he had just had his insides ripped out he might expect you to take on more household duties. I am positive you will be a happier person with a higher self esteem when you are able to fit into some of your clothes. You can't lose sight of yourself now. Motherhood is a very selfless job. If you let your physical fitness go now, you won't be happy about it in the long run. Hire someone to clean the house. You can't hire someone to sleep or workout for you. A dirty house can be cleaned up in a few hours, a day or two if it's a big house. You can't get a great figure in a day. Let the house go, not your figure. Seriously, you are worth every second you spend exercising and raising your self esteem. I know very few people who have high self esteem because their house was clean and dinner was on the table for the two months after they gave birth. I know a lot of my training clients have very high self esteem because they look better than ever and their house is clean now, so who cares!

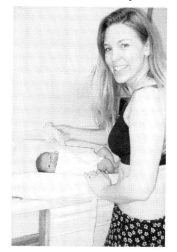

7 days postpartum
No makeup, no highlights, no shirt

2-3 Weeks Postpartum

Add these activities:

- Postpartum bleeding, even for women who have had a C-section, usually lasts for two to three weeks after delivery. For some women, it can last up to eight weeks. Once bleeding has stopped, you should return to your third trimester workout schedule. Your third trimester workout schedule should be perfect for postpartum recovery, because it involves no jarring movements, no jumping, very light weight and shorter, more frequent cardio sessions. You will be following your fitness footsteps in reverse, with the goal of starting your first trimester workout schedule after your six week postpartum checkup. As long as you are healthy and healing well, you can progress in terms of performance back through your second trimester over the next four weeks. That is, try to gain speed, duration, intensity and exercise difficulty so that when you hit six weeks postpartum, your fitness level will be equivalent to your fitness level at 13 weeks pregnant. I don't expect you to be able to perform as well as you did during your first trimester, I just want you conditioned enough that you can drag yourself through your old first trimester workouts. This timeline is realistic if you exercised up until your due date. Adjust your personal timeline based on when you stop bleeding and how fit you currently are. This sounds like a fast transition, but remember, you are already about ten pounds lighter without the baby and placenta and you are not pregnant, so you can breathe and move much easier. Plus, you are stronger after doing the Mommy Fabulous Program while pregnant.

- Great Mommy Fabulous abdominal recovery exercises are any and all balancing moves because they target the core. All kicks and leg lifts performed very slowly with total control are appropriate, but you may not be able to kick as high depending on perineal soreness.

- Begin twisting and torso rotation exercises. The Mommy Fabulous abs exercises are great. They are targeted at pulling the waist in tight.

- Sit on a body ball while holding your baby to your chest. Lean back in a pelvic tilt and perform ball crunches.

6 Weeks Postpartum
Add these activities:

- At six weeks postpartum you should receive the green light from your healthcare provider to return to all normal activities. This means you should return to your first trimester workout regimen. If you did Step, Spin, Cycling or Kickboxing you should return to class and be capable of anywhere from 50-80% of your performance during your first trimester. You should return to your first trimester Mommy Fabulous weightlifting program, but not necessarily be capable of the same dumbbell weight or exercise difficulty you were capable of in the first trimester. You will still have the effects of pregnancy hormones in your system for up to five months, so you will continue to be careful about joint laxity if you are going to return to a sport. Returning to moderately paced tennis practice is more appropriate than returning to competitive matches at this point.

- You may want to get on a scale, just to see how far you have to go. Beware! I feel that when my clients are focused on weight they tend to feel more depressed about it. When their waist is shrinking and looking more defined they are not celebrating because their weight hasn't budged.

- Performing speed drills between weightlifting sets greatly increases weight loss. This is called interval training and is far more effective for weight loss than traditional cardio.

- Wearing your baby in a front carrier while doing sumo squats can be great exercise at home.

- Until your baby is sleeping through the night you need to continue to take naps. It is not lazy! It is part of your weight loss program!!!!

- If you are returning to work, you need to realize that your recovery isn't over. There are going to be more demands on you, but you need to be one of your top priorities. Six weeks of leave isn't enough. You may not be bleeding anymore, but your body has not recovered. Practice as much of the above advise as you can while at work and nap as much as you can on weekends.

4 Months Postpartum
Add these activities:

- If you gained an appropriate amount of weight according to Chapter Seven, you should probably be back to your pre-pregnancy weight around month four or five. If you had multiple babies, it may take longer. You probably won't be able to shed the last five pounds while nursing because of the weight of the breast tissue and due to the hormones involved in lactation. I am not too concerned about numbers. Do you like the way you look?

- If you have lost the pregnancy weight, you may notice that if you flex your abs, you have a flat stomach, but if you don't, it still has a tendency to sag outward. You will have to be mindful to hold your abs to support your posture for a few more months before they are trained to stay tight. You may also notice that even if your stomach is almost there, you still have extra skin. If you a grab a chunk of it, it will feel empty, not like grabbing a chunk of fat. It will take between six months and one year post delivery for the skin to shrink back to the size of your new tiny abdomen. Likewise, it may take up to six months for a linea negra to disappear.

- Think about the way you move outside the gym. You should be doing tons of squats! Your baby should be doing lots of floor time to increase strength for rolling over and crawling. Are you doing a sumo squat every time you pick your baby up off the floor? If you are on the floor, what muscles and technique do you use to get up? When you need to set something down on the floor, do it as a reverse lunge. If you find yourself bending over a lot, try to pretend you are in public, in the tiniest mini skirt. Don't avoid the constant opportunity for exercise and calorie burning that motherhood provides by bending over.

- Challenge yourself over the next two months. If you started this book as a Beginner, try to push yourself toward Intermediate fitness.

6 Months Postpartum

- Hormones and any lasting effects on joints should be back to normal unless you are still breastfeeding.

- Fitness should be 100% recovered to pre-pregnancy levels if not better.

- If you followed the program, your body should look better than ever. If you want to lose more weight, or get into even better shape, go for it!

The Big Picture

Don't let postpartum recovery become an obsession that gets you down. This program is exactly what I did and when I did it, but it should be used as a guide, not as a basis for judging yourself. If you are not quite where you want to be six months later, guess what, you still have plenty of time. Don't get desperate and please don't turn to a terrible fad diet that will ruin your metabolism and everything you have worked for. Fad diets rarely if ever provide weight loss that is life long. People usually end up yo-yoing. Being healthy, happy and fit is what Mommy Fabulous is about; it's a lifestyle and a mindset. I think you are a fantastic mom who should take the time and effort it takes to make you feel and look as amazing as you are. Good luck and enjoy being Mommy Fabulous!

Acknowledgments

Writing a book is a bit like raising a child. It takes a village of people who carefully advise, encourage and support throughout the journey. My goal was to write a book providing all the information needed to minimize the complications of pregnancy and provide a physical therapy based fitness program that speeds up postpartum recovery time safely. Getting it published was really secondary. The fact that it is currently available is due to numerous people in my village, all of whom I would like to thank.

I am very grateful to have a wonderful family who champions every endeavor I undertake. My parents are always my greatest source of encouragement and my biggest fans. I appreciate my brother bragging about me to all his friends. I owe acknowledgement to Devin Giannoni, my PR Director. Devin was my sound board, making priceless suggestions on tone and content. Thank you for putting pressure on me to finish and guiding me on branding, media and marketing. Without the public relations savvy of my sister Devin, I would not have known where to start. Her photography skills shaped a large portion of the book and she has done an amazing job publicizing Mommy Fabulous.

Thanks to my pregnant and postpartum clients who contributed to this book by sharing their experiences, questions and concerns about exercise and nutrition. Thank you Judy Crosby for taking the time to do a first-pass editing; this book has come a long way! I owe a huge debt of gratitude to Jordan Giannoni for the professional editing that made all the difference in bringing this project to its current polished status. I have had several supporters who have provided essential encouragement and nagging as deadlines have loomed and arrived. A heart felt thank you goes to Marla Livengood who was one of my first pregnant readers of the nearly completed manuscript who applied the principals. Thanks for telling me for nearly a year afterward how helpful the book was. The fact you have read every book in the prenatal category and strongly felt Mommy Fabulous provided more essential advice meant a lot. Your insistence that this information should be available to all women has kept me from leaving the completed manuscript in the closet.

Last, but certainly not least, I am deeply grateful for my husband, Mike. It was through his love and support that I had the time and resources to give this project the attention and effort it required. He is my life partner, my exercise partner and my rock. I love you.

Danielle Federico, M.P.H.
October 2011

Sources

1. Organization of Teratology Information Services (OTIS): Toxoplasmosis Pregnancy. January 2007 <http://otispregnancy.org/pdf/toxoplasmosis.pdf> Retrieved February 2009.
2. Food and Drug Administration (FDA), Center for Food Safety and Applied Nutrition. Growing Sprouts in Retail Food Establishments. CFP Issues 02- III - 01 and 04 –III-012. December 2004. < http://www.foodsafety.gov/keep/types/fruits/sprouts.html > Retrieved February 2012.
3. Food and Drug Administration (FDA), Center for Food Safety and Applied Nutrition: Safe Handling of Raw Produce and Fresh Squeezed Fruit and Vegetables. < http://www.foodsafety.gov/keep/types/fruits/tipsfreshprodsafety.html> Retrieved February 2012.
4. Organization of Teratology Information Services (OTIS): Methelmercury and Pregnancy. October 2004. <http://otispregnancy.org/pdf/methylmercury.pdf> Retrieved February 2009.
5. US Department of Health and Human Services and the US Environmental Protection Agency: Mercury Levels in Commercial Fish and Shellfish, Updated February 2012. <http://sis.nlm.nih.gov/enviro/mercury.html> Retrieved February 2012.
6. Weng, X., et al: Maternal Caffeine Consumption during Pregnancy and the Risk of Miscarriage: A Prospective Cohort Study. American Journal of Obstetrics and Gynecology, published online, January 21, 2008. Retrieved February 2009.
7. Organization of Teratology Information Services (OTIS): Caffeine and Pregnancy. December 2006. <http://otispregnancy.org/pdf/caffeine.pdf> Retrieved February 2009.
8. Institute of Medicine. Food and Nutrition Board: Dietary Reference Intakes for Vitamin A, Vitamin K, Arsenic, Boron, Chromium, Copper, Iodine, Iron, Manganese, Molybdenum, Nickel, Silicon, Vanadium and Zinc. Washington, DC: National Academy Press, 2001.
9. American Academy of Pediatrics, Committee on Drugs. Policy Statement: The Transfer of Drugs and Other Chemicals into Human Milk. Pediatrics, September 2001; 108 (3): 776-789.
10. Chart compiled with information from <http://www.rockstar69.com/products.php>; <http://otispregnancy.org/pdf/caffeine.pdf> <http://www.hersheys.com/nutrition/caffeine.asp><www.starbucks.com> Retrieved April 2009.
11. Malik, S., et al: Maternal Smoking and Congenital Heart Defects. Pediatrics, April 2008; 121 (4): e810-e816.
12. Law, K.L., et al: Smoking During Pregnancy and Newborn Neurobehavior. Pediatrics, June 2003; 111 (6): 1318-1323.
13. March of Dimes: Smoking During Pregnancy. April 2008. <http://www.marchofdimes.com/professionals/14332_1171.asp> Retrieved February 2009.
14. The American College of Obstetricians and Gynecologists (ACOG): Your Pregnancy & Birth, Fourth Edition, 2005.
15. Mohr C: The Dangers of High Fructose Corn Syrup Is This Disguised Sugar Affecting Your Diabetes? Diabetes Health, May 2005.
16. The Independent: Deadly fats: why are we still eating them? June 10, 2008. Retrieved June 2008.
17. Pressinger R, Project Supervisor - Marfo K University of South Florida Special Education Department: Environmental Causes of Learning Disabilities and Child Neurological Disorders, Review of Research. < http://chem-tox.com/pregnancy/learning_disabilities.htm?vm=r > Retrieved May 2009.
18. US Dept of Agriculture: Why is it important to eat grains, especially whole grains? Last Modified: March 13 2009. < http://www.choosemyplate.gov/food-groups/grains-why.html > Retrieved Feb 20112.
19. Kovacs B: Artificial Sweeteners MedicineNet, Inc. < http://www.medicinenet.com/artificial_sweeteners/page10.htm >Retrieved April, 2009.
20. Swithers S, Davidson T: A Role for Sweet Taste: Calorie Predictive Relations in Energy Regulation by Rats (PDF: 675KB). Behavioral Neuroscience, February 2008.
21. Mennella JA, Jagnow CP, Beauchamp GK: Prenatal and postnatal flavor learning by human infants. Pediatrics, 2001 Jun;107(6):E88.
22. Dounchis, J.Z., Hayden, H.A., & Wilfley, D.E.: Obesity, eating disorders, and body image in ethnically diverse children and adolescents. In J.K. Thompson and L. Smolak (Eds.) Body Image, Eating Disorders, and Obesity in Children and Adolescents: Theory, Assessment, Treatment, & Prevention. Washington, D.C.: American Psychological Association (2001).
23. Hyattsville MD: U.S. Department of Health and Human Services, Centers for Disease Control and Prevention, National Center for Health Statistics: Prevalence of Overweight Among Children and Adolescents: United States, 1999-2002 This page last reviewed Sept. 9, 2008. < http://www.cdc.gov/nchs/products/pubs/pubd/hestats/overwght99.htm> Retrieved April 2009.
24. U.S. Department of Agriculture, Center for Nutrition Policy and Promotion: Where do your favorite foods fit in? Dietary Guidelines For Americans Putting the Guidelines into Practice. Feb 2003 http://www.pueblo.gsa.gov/cic_text/food/fav-food/fav.htm Retrieved April 2009.
25. California Avocado Commission: Approved California Avocado Nutrition Copy Points as of 6/6/07. Retrieved April 21, 2009.
26. European Journal of Obstetrics, Gynecology & Reproductive Biology, 1990, vol.38
27. The National Digestive Diseases Information Clearinghouse: http://www.digestive.niddk.nih.gov/ NIH Publication No. 07–2754. July 2007. Retrieved April 2009.
28. Gelfand J (reviewed by) Web MD: Frequently Asked Questions About Food Triggers, Migraines, and Headaches. Last reviewed on January 23. http://www.webmd.com/migraines-headaches/guide/triggers-specific-foods Retrieved April 2009.
29. March of Dimes: Foundation Headaches. 2009. www.marchofdimes.com Retrieved April 2009.
30. Institute of Medicine, Food and Nutrition Board: Dietary Reference Intakes for Vitamin A, Vitamin K, Arsenic, Boron, Chromium, Copper, Iodine, Iron, Manganese, Molybdenum, Nickel, Silicon, Vanadium and Zinc. Washington, DC: National Academy Press, 2001.
31. Jovanovic L, American Diabetes Association's Fourth International Workshop: conference on gestational diabetes mellitus: summary and discussion. Therapeutic Interventions. 1998;21(suppl 2);B131–7.
32. American Pregnancy Association. Pregnancy Nutrition. November 2008. <http://www.americanpregnancy.org/pregnancyhealth/pregnancynutrition.html> Retrieved February 2009.
33. Hillier, Teresa, et al: Gaining Too Much Weight During Pregnancy Nearly Doubles Risk of Having A Heavy Baby. Obstetrics & Gynecology 2008.
34. National Heart, Lung and Blood Institute. Adapted from Clinical Guidelines on the Identification, Evaluation and Treatment of Overweight and Obesity in Adults: The Evidence Report. U.S. Department of Health and Human Services, 1998.
35. Artal R: Editorial comments. Expert Review of Obstetrics and Gynecology. March 2008. https://www.slu.edu/x21566.xml Retrieved May 2009.
36. Martin J, Hamilton B, et al; CDC Division of Vital Statistics: National Vital Statistics Report Volume 54, Number 2 September 8, 2005 Births: Final Data for 2003.
37. American College of Obstetricians and Gynecologists (ACOG): Intrauterine Growth Restriction. ACOG Practice Bulletin, number 12, January 2000.

38. American Pregnancy Association. Most Common Pregnancy Complications. April 2006.
<http://www.americanpregnancy.org/pregnancycomplications/commoncomplications.html > Retrieved February 2009.

39. Boulé NG, Haddad E, Kenny GP, Wells GA, Sigal RJ: Effects of exercise on glycemic control and body mass in type 2 diabetes mellitus: a meta-analysis of controlled clinical trials. JAMA. 2001 Sep 12;286(10):1218-27.

40. March of Dimes, Pregnancy and Health Education Center: Weight gain during pregnancy. February 2008.
<http://www.marchofdimes.com/pnhec/159_153.asp> Retrieved February 2009.

41. Wallace AM, Boyer DB, Dan A, et al: Aerobic exercise, maternal self-esteem, and physical discomforts during pregnancy. J Nurse Midwife 1986; 31 (6):255-262.

42. American Diabetes Association: Gestational Diabetes. <http://www.diabetes.org/gestational-diabetes.jsp> Retrieved February 2009.

43. Wolfe LA, Hall P, Webb KA, et al: Prescription of aerobic exercise during pregnancy. Sports Med 1989; 8(5):273-301.

44. Clapp JF III: The course of labor after endurance exercise during pregnancy. Am J Obstet Gynecol 1990; 163(6 pt1): 1799-1805.

45. Wang TW; Apgar BS: Exercise during pregnancy. Am Fam Physician 1998; 57(8): 1846-52.

46. Hall DC, Kaufmann DA: Effects of aerobic and strength conditioning on pregnancy outcomes. *Am J Obstet Gynecol.* 1987;157:1199-1203.

47. Downs DS, Hausenblas HA: Exercising for two: examining pregnant women's second trimester exercise intention and behavior using the framework of the theory of planned behavior. *Women's Health Issues.* 2003;13:222-228.

48. Clapp, J.F: Influence of Endurance Exercise and Diet on Human Placental Development and Fetal Growth. Placenta, June-July 2006; 27: 527-534.

49. American College of Sports Medicine. Roundtable Consensus Statement: Impact of Physical Activity During Pregnancy and Postpartum on Chronic Disease Risk. Medicine and Science in Sports and Exercise, 2006; vol pg 989-1005.

50. Clapp JF 3d: The changing thermal response to endurance exercise during pregnancy. Am J Obstet Gynecol 1991;165:1684-9.

51. Stevenson L: Exercise in pregnancy: part 2: recommendations for individuals. Can Fam Physician 1997;43(1):107-111.

52. Organization of Teratology Information Services (OTIS): Hyperthermia and Pregnancy. July 2006, <http://otispregnancy.org/pdf/hyperthermia.pdf > Retrieved May 2009

53. American College of Obstetricians and Gynecologists (ACOG): Exercise During Pregnancy. Education Pamphlet Number AP119. June 2003, updated 2009.

54. Artal R, Platt L, Sperling M, et al: Exercise in pregnancy, Maternal cardiovascular ad metabolic responses in normal pregnancy. American Journal of Obstetrics and Gynecology 1981; 140:123.

55. Clapp, J.F.,III: Recommending Exercise during Pregnancy. Contemporary Ob/Gyn, January 2001: 30-49.

56. Artal R, O'Toole M: Guidelines of the American College of Obstetricians and Gynecologists for exercise during pregnancy and the postpartum period. January <http://www.ncbi.nlm.nih.gov/pmc/articles/PMC1724598/ > Retrieved Feb 2012.

57. Karzel RP, Friedman MJ: Orthopedic injuries in pregnancy. In: Artal R, Wiswell RA, Drinkwater BL, eds. Exercise in pregnancy. 2nd ed. Baltimore: Williams and Wilkins, 1991.

58. American College of Obstetricians and Gynecologists (ACOG): Exercise during pregnancy and the postpartum period. Technical Bulletin Number 189—February 1994. Int J Gynaecol Obstet 1994;45(1):65-70.

59. Calguneri M, Bird HA, Wright V: Changes in joint laxity occurring during pregnancy. Ann Rheum Dis 1982;41(2):126-128.

60. Branstrom, MA: Clinical Kinesiology, 3rd ed., F.A. Davis, Philadelphia, 1981.

61. Presidents Council for Physical Fitness and Sports: Guidelines for Personal Exercise Programs pamphlet 2009, last updated on 03/13/2009 http://www.fitness.gov/fitness.pdf Retrieved May 2009.

62. McCrory MA, Nommsen-Rivers LA, Mole PA, et al: Randomized trial of short-term effects of dieting compared with dieting plus aerobic exercise on lactation performance. Am J Clin Nutr 1999;69:959–67.

Made in the USA
Lexington, KY
31 October 2013